AF821056

Oncology

International Journal of Cancer Research and Treatment

Founded 1948 as 'Oncologia' by H.R. Schinz
Continued by V. Richards (1967–1975), H. Wrba (1976–1992), P.P. Carbone (1993–2002), D.L. Trump (2002–2007)

KARGER

Printed in Switzerland
on acid-free and non-aging
paper (ISO 9706) by
Reinhardt Druck, Basel

Appears monthly:
2 volumes per year
(12 issues)

Oncology

Guidelines for Authors

Submission

Original papers and reviews written in English are considered for publication. **Manuscripts should be submitted to 'Oncology' online.** For specific instructions on how to prepare a manuscript for submission, you are encouraged to view the guidelines at **www.karger.com/ocl**, where you will also find a link to the **Submission Website**. Names, postal and e-mail addresses of at least four experts in the appropriate area of research must accompany each manuscript. Selected scientists will be invited to act as referees. Referees suggested should not be from the same institution as the author and should have expert knowledge of the subject. Should you have any problems with your submission, please contact:

Dr. M. Markman
S. Karger AG
Editorial Office 'Oncology'
CH–4009 Basel (Switzerland)
Tel. +41 61 306 1359
Fax +41 61 306 1434
E-Mail ocl@karger.com

Mailing address for courier deliveries only:
Allschwilerstr. 10
CH–4055 Basel (Switzerland)

Conditions

All manuscripts are subject to editorial review. Manuscripts are received with the explicit understanding that they are not under simultaneous consideration by any other publication. The editors reserve the right to improve style and, if necessary, return the manuscript for rewriting to the author. Submission of an article for publication implies the transfer of the copyright from the author to the publisher upon acceptance. Accepted papers become the permanent property of 'Oncology' and may not be reproduced by any means, in whole or in part, without the written consent of the publisher. It is the author's responsibility to obtain permission to reproduce illustrations, tables, etc. from other publications.
All manuscripts originating from non-English speaking countries must be revised by a professional linguistic reviewer and it must be evident from the covering letter that this has been done.
The editor reserves the right to reject papers based on priorities and space availability in the journal.

Conflicts of Interest

Authors are required to disclose any sponsorship or funding arrangements relating to their research and all authors should disclose any possible conflicts of interest. Conflict of interest statements will be published at the end of the text of the article.

Ethical and Legal Prerequisites

Manuscripts involving examinations of human subjects must include a statement that the trial protocol has been approved by an ethical committee and thus meets the standards of the Declaration of Helsinki in its revised version of 1975 and its amendments of 1983, 1989, and 1996 [JAMA 1997;277:925–926]. Accordingly, the subject's informed consent has to be mentioned in the manuscript. Information suitable to reveal the subject's identity is to be avoided.

Categories of Manuscripts

Reviews are comprehensive, state-of-the-art analyses and investigations of important clinical problems. Reviews must include a critical discussion of the reported data and give a clear conclusion with the potential impacts on the standard of care. Reviews may be invited by the Editor, or they may be unsolicited submissions. Reviews are not subject to page charges. The maximum length of manuscripts in this category will be 5,000 words for text and tables (a table = 250 words per page), with a maximum of 5 tables and 50 references.

Clinical Studies and *Clinical Translational Research Articles* are full-length research papers which will be considered for the journal. These articles cover topics relevant to clinical and translational studies in all oncological fields. Note that manuscripts presenting laboratory-based research efforts must address a clinically relevant issue (Translational Research).

Short Communications will focus on descriptions of important toxicities of novel therapies and highly unique oncology-related medical management issues. The maximum length of manuscripts in this category will be 1,000 words.

Clinical Trial Notes are designed for brief discussions of clinical trials, with a particular focus on phase 1, phase 1/2, and phase 2 studies. Priority in this section will not be for studies with a 'positive result', but rather for well-conceived and conducted clinical research efforts. The maximum length of manuscripts submitted in this category will be 1,500 words, with a maximum of 2 tables and 1 figure. The paper should be divided into four sections: Introduction, Methods, Results, Discussion. Note that all manuscripts submitted in this category will undergo rapid review for acceptance or rejection.

Reducing the Worldwide Burden of Cancer are country reports describing a variety of regional, national or international efforts that focus on the unique aspects of the epidemiology of cancer, and the delivery of educational messages, preventive services, and oncology-related care within the developing world. Papers submitted for this section benefit from a higher quota of free pages. There are no page charges for papers of 8 or fewer printed pages. Each additional complete or partial page is charged to the author at CHF 325.00.

Editorials are commentaries on current topics or on papers published elsewhere in the issue. Word count limit is 1500 and 10 references are allowed. They are usually invited by the Editor.

Letters addressed *to the Editor* are encouraged if they directly concern articles previously published in this journal and clinical subjects related to the matters discussed. The editor reserves the right to submit copies of such letters to the authors of the articles concerned prior to publication in order to permit them to respond in the same issue of the journal. But letters on general scientific or medical subjects in oncology are also welcome. The length should not exceed 500 words.

Arrangement

Title page: The first page of each paper should indicate the title, the authors' names, the institute where the work was conducted, and a short title for use as running head.

Full address: The exact postal address of the corresponding author complete with postal code must be given at the bottom of the title page. Please also supply phone and fax numbers, as well as e-mail address.

Key words: Please supply 3–10 key words in English that reflect the content of the paper.

Abstract: Papers submitted to the sections Reviews, Clinical Studies, Clinical Translational Research Articles, Clinical Trial Notes and Reducing the Worldwide Burden of Cancer need an abstract of up to 200 words. Abstracts are recommended, but optional, for Short Communications and Editorials. Abstracts of papers submitted for publication that have clinical implications using human materials should be structured with subheadings as follows: Objective(s), Methods, Results, Conclusion(s).

Footnotes: Avoid footnotes. When essential, they are numbered consecutively and typed at the foot of the appropriate page.

Tables and illustrations: Tables and illustrations (both numbered in Arabic numerals) should be prepared on separate pages. Tables require a heading and figures a legend, also prepared on a separate page. Due to technical reasons, figures with a screen background should not be submitted. When possible, group several illustrations in one block for reproduction (max. size 180 × 223 mm) or provide crop marks. Each illustration must be labelled with its number and the first author's name. B/w half-tone and color illustrations must have a final resolution of 300 dpi after scaling, line drawings one of 800–1,200 dpi. Figure files must not be embedded in a document file but submitted separately (see detailed instructions on the Submission Website at **www.karger.com/ocl**).

Color illustrations
Online edition: Color illustrations are reproduced free of charge. In the print version, the illustrations are reproduced in black and white. Please avoid referring to the colors in the text and figure legends.
Print edition: Up to 6 color illustrations per page can be integrated within the text at CHF 800.– per page.

References

In the text identify references by Arabic numerals [in square brackets]. Material submitted for publication but not yet accepted should be noted as 'unpublished data' and not be included in the reference list. The list of references should include only those publications which are cited in the text. Do not alphabetize; number references in the order in which they are first mentioned in the text. The surnames of the authors followed by initials should be given. There should be no punctuation other than a comma to separate the authors. Preferably, please cite all authors. Abbreviate journal names according to the Index Medicus system. Also see International Committee of Medical Journal Editors: Uniform requirements for manuscripts submitted to biomedical journals (www.icmje.org).

KARGER
E-Mail karger@karger.com
www.karger.com

The Guidelines for Authors are available at:
www.karger.com/ocl_Guidelines

Examples
(a) Papers published in periodicals: Chatel J-M, Bernard H, Orson FM: Isolation and characterization of two complete Ara h 2 isoforms cDNA. Int Arch Allergy Immunol 2003;131:14–18.
(b) Papers published only with DOI numbers: Theoharides TC, Boucher W, Spear K: Serum interleukin-6 reflects disease severity and osteoporosis in mastocytosis patients. Int Arch Allergy Immunol DOI: 10.1159/000063858.
(c) Monographs: Matthews DE, Farewell VT: Using and Understanding Medical Statistics, ed 3, revised. Basel, Karger, 1996.0
(d) Edited books: Cochrane AL, Ricardo SD: Oxidant stress and regulation of chemokines in the development of renal interstitial fibrosis; in Razzaque MS, Taguchi T (eds): Renal Fibrosis. Contrib Nephrol. Basel, Karger, 2003, vol 139, pp 102–119.
Reference Management Software: Use of EndNote is recommended for easy management and formatting of citations and reference lists.

Digital Object Identifier (DOI)
S. Karger Publishers supports DOIs as unique identifiers for articles. A DOI number will be printed on the title page of each article. DOIs can be useful in the future for identifying and citing articles published online without volume or issue information. More information can be found at www.doi.org.

Supplementary Material
Supplementary material is restricted to additional data that are not necessary for the scientific integrity and conclusions of the paper. Please note that all supplementary files will undergo editorial review and should be submitted together with the original manuscript. The Editors reserve the right to limit the scope and length of the supplementary material. Supplementary material must meet production quality standards for Web publication without the need for any modification or editing. In general, supplementary files should not exceed 10 MB in size. All figures and tables should have titles and legends and all files should be supplied separately and named clearly. Acceptable files and formats are: Word or PDF files, Excel spreadsheets (only if the data cannot be converted properly to a PDF file), and video files (.mov, .avi, .mpeg).

Author's Choice™
Karger's Author's Choice™ service broadens the reach of your article and gives all users worldwide free and full access for reading, downloading and printing at www.karger.com. The option is available for a one-time fee of CHF 3000.–, which is a permissible cost in grant allocation. More information can be found at www.karger.com/authors_choice.

NIH-Funded Research
The U.S. National Institutes of Health (NIH) mandates under the NIH Public Access Policy that final, peer-reviewed manuscripts appear in its digital database within 12 months of the official publication date. As a service to authors, Karger submits the final version of your article on your behalf to PubMed Central. For those selecting our premium Author's Choice™ service, we will send your article immediately upon publishing, accelerating the accessibility of your work without the usual embargo. More details on NIH's Public Access Policy is available at http://publicaccess.nih.gov/policy.htm

Self-Archiving
Karger permits authors to archive their pre-prints (i.e. pre-refereeing) or post-prints (i.e. final draft post-refereeing) on their personal or institution's servers, provided the following conditions are met: Articles may not be used for commercial purposes, must be linked to the publisher's version, and must acknowledge the publisher's copyright. Authors selecting Karger's Author's Choice™ feature, however, are also permitted to archive the final, published version of their article, which includes copyediting and design improvements as well as citation links.

Page Charges
There are no page charges for papers of 3 or fewer printed pages (including tables, illustrations and references). Each additional complete or partial page is charged to the author at CHF 325.–. The allotted size of a paper is equal to approx. 9 manuscript pages (including tables, illustrations and references).

Proofs
Unless indicated otherwise, proofs are sent to the corresponding author and should be returned with the least possible delay. Alterations other than the correction of printer's errors are charged to the author.

Reprints
Order forms and a price list are sent with the proofs. Orders submitted after the issue is printed are subject to considerably higher prices.

KARGER

E-Mail karger@karger.com
www.karger.com

The Guidelines for Authors are available at:
www.karger.com/ocl_Guidelines

Oncology

General Information

ISSN Print Edition: 0030–2414
ISSN Online Edition: 1423–0232

Journal Homepage: www.karger.com/ocl

Publication Data: 'Oncology' is published 12 times a year. Volumes 84 and 85, each with 6 issues, appear in 2013.

Subscription Rates: Subscriptions run for a full calendar year. Prices are given per year.
Personal subscription:

Print or Online	Print+Online combined
CHF 1622.–	CHF 1718.–
EUR 1308.–	EUR 1386.–
USD 1606.00	USD 1702.00

postage and handling (added to print and print+online)
CHF 86.40 Europe, CHF 124.80 Overseas
EUR 67.20
USD 115.20

Institutional subscription:

Print or Online	Print+Online combined
CHF 3244.–	CHF 3568.–
EUR 2616.–	EUR 2878.–
USD 3212.00	USD 3532.00

postage and handling (added to print and print+online)
CHF 108.– Europe, CHF 156.– Overseas
EUR 84.–
USD 144.00

Airmail surcharge: CHF 105.– / USD 99.00

Back Volumes and Single Issues: Information on availability and prices of single print issues and print or electronic back volumes can be obtained from Customer Service at *service@karger.com.*

Bibliographic Indices: This journal is regularly listed in bibliographic services, including *Current Contents®* and PubMed/MEDLINE.

Photocopying: This journal has been registered with the Copyright Clearance Center (CCC), as indicated by the code appearing on the first page of each article. For readers in the US, this code signals consent for copying of articles for personal or internal use, or for the personal or internal use of specific clients, provided that the stated fee is paid per copy directly to
Copyright Clearance Center Inc.
222 Rosewood Drive
Danvers, MA 01923 (USA)
A copy of the first page of the article must accompany payment. Consent does not extend to copying for general distribution, for promotion, for creating new works, or for resale. In these cases, specific written permission must be obtained from the copyright owner,
S. Karger AG, P.O. Box
CH–4009 Basel (Switzerland).

Subscription Orders:
Orders can be placed at agencies, bookstores, directly with the Publisher

S. Karger AG
Medical and Scientific Publishers
Allschwilerstrasse 10
CH–4009 Basel
Switzerland

t: +41 61 306 11 11
f: +41 61 306 12 34
e: karger@karger.com
w: www.karger.com

(for courier services only:
Allschwilerstrasse 10
CH–4055 Basel)

or further Karger offices or representatives:

Germany
S. Karger GmbH
Postfach
79095 Freiburg
Deutschland
(Hausadresse: Wilhelmstrasse 20A, 79098 Freiburg)
t: +49 761 45 20 70
f: +49 761 45 20 714
e: information@karger.de
w: www.karger.de

Japan
Karger Japan, Inc.
Shiba Daimon Asahi Bldg. 2F
1-2-23 Shiba Daimon
Minato-ku
Tokyo 105-0012
Japan
t: +81 3 6435 6242
f: +81 3 6435 6244
e: publisher@karger.jp
w: www.karger.jp

USA
S. Karger Publishers, Inc.
26 West Avon Road
P.O. Box 529
Unionville, CT 06085
USA
Toll free: +1 800 828 5479
t: +1 860 675 7834
f: +1 860 675 7302
e: karger@snet.net

France
Librairie Médi-Sciences Sarl
36, bd de Latour-Maubourg
75007 Paris
France
t: +33 (0) 1 45 51 42 58
f: +33 (0) 1 45 56 07 80
e: librairie@medi-sciences.fr
w: www.medi-sciences.fr

South East Asia, China and Taiwan
Karger Regional Office (Malaysia)
CEO Suite Kuala Lumpur
Quill 7, 27th Floor
Jalan Stesen Sentral 5
KL Sentral
Kuala Lumpur 50470
Malaysia
t: +60 3 2776 6803
f: +60 3 2776 6999
e: service@karger.cn; r.chew@karger.cn

Karger China
10th Floor, Twin Towers (East)
B12 Jianguomenwai Avenue
Beijing 100022
China
t: +86 10 5123 5033
f: +86 10 5123 5122
e: service@karger.cn; r.chew@karger.cn
w: www.karger.cn

India, Bangladesh, Sri Lanka
Medscience India
Plot No. 17, Yusuf Sarai Market
B.L. Glass Building, 2nd Floor
Sri Aurobindo Marg
New Delhi 110 016
India
t: +91 11 46029 633
f: +91 11 46029 634
c: +91 98 91052 128
e: medsci.india@gmail.com

Change of Address:
Both old and new address should be sent to the subscription source.

The Guidelines for Authors are available at:
www.karger.com/ocl_Guidelines

Oncology

The 3rd Asia-Pacific Primary Liver Cancer Expert Meeting

July 6–8, 2012, Shanghai, China

The 48th Annual Meeting of the Liver Cancer Study Group of Japan

July 20–21, 2012, Kanazawa, Japan

Guest Editors
Kwang-Hyub Han, Seoul
Masatoshi Kudo, Osaka
Sheng-Long Ye, Shanghai

25 figures, 5 in color, and 16 tables, 2013

KARGER

Basel · Freiburg · Paris · London · New York · New Delhi · Bangkok · Beijing · Tokyo · Kuala Lumpur · Singapore · Sydney

Disclosure Statement Guest Editors

The editors declare that no conflicts of interests exist.

S. Karger
Medical and Scientific Publishers
Basel · Freiburg · Paris · London · New York ·
New Delhi · Bangkok · Beijing · Tokyo ·
Kuala Lumpur · Singapore · Sydney

Disclaimer
The statements, opinions and data contained in this publication are solely those of the individual authors and contributors and not of the publisher and the editor(s). The appearance of advertisements in the journal is not a warranty, endorsement, or approval of the products or services advertised or of their effectiveness, quality or safety. The publisher and the editor(s) disclaim responsibility for any injury to persons or property resulting from any ideas, methods, instructions or products referred to in the content or advertisements.

Drug Dosage
The authors and the publisher have exerted every effort to ensure that drug selection and dosage set forth in this text are in accord with current recommendations and practice at the time of publication. However, in view of ongoing research, changes in government regulations, and the constant flow of information relating to drug therapy and drug reactions, the reader is urged to check the package insert for each drug for any change in indications and dosage and for added warnings and precautions. This is particularly important when the recommended agent is a new and/or infrequently employed drug.

P.O. Box, CH–4009 Basel (Switzerland)
Printed in Switzerland
on acid-free and non-aging paper (ISO 9706) by
Reinhardt Druck, Basel
ISBN 978–3–318–02334–3
e-ISBN 978–3–318–02335–0

KARGER

E-Mail karger@karger.com

Vol. 84, Suppl. 1, 2013

Oncology

Contents

KARGER

E-Mail karger@karger.com

Access to full text and tables of contents, including tentative ones for forthcoming issues: www.karger.com/ocl_issues

Preface

Oncology

Oncology 2013;84(suppl 1):1–2
DOI: 10.1159/000345882

Published online: February 20, 2013

Advances in Liver Fibrosis Imaging and Hepatocellular Carcinoma: Update in 2013

Masatoshi Kudo

Kinki University School of Medicine, Osakasayama, Japan

The 3rd Asia-Pacific Primary Liver Cancer Expert Meeting (APPLE) was held on July 6–8, 2012, in Shanghai, China. In this meeting more than 50 invited international speakers and more than 500 participants from Asian countries participated. Highly scientific lectures followed by active discussion made this meeting an invaluable one.

The 48th Annual Meeting of the Liver Cancer Study Group of Japan was held on July 20–21, 2012, in Kanazawa, Japan. This meeting was also active and outstanding. This supplement issue contains selected articles with a high scientific value from these 2 meetings.

Fujimoto et al. [1] and Yada et al. [2] describe the usefulness of noninvasive techniques in evaluating liver fibrosis using real-time tissue elastography (RTE). RTE is a strain elastography in contrast to shear wave elastography in the diagnosis of liver stiffness. According to these 2 articles, RTE seems to be a promising method in evaluating liver fibrosis stage.

Kudo et al. [3] describe the role of gadolinum-ethoxybenzyl-diethylenetriamine imaging (Gd-EOB-DTPA MRI) in the management of hepatocellular carcinoma (HCC). This is a report based on the votes cast by 144 HCC experts at the 48th Annual Meeting of the Liver Cancer Study Group of Japan. The voting results which achieved more than 67% agreement are summarized as 'consensus statements'. Furthermore, issues which obtained more than 50% agreement are summarized as 'informative statements'. This report presents very interesting results and reflects daily clinical practice on use of EOB-MRI in Japan.

Takayasu [4] contributes a state-of-the-art article on transcatheter arterial chemoembolization (TACE) for unresectable HCC. The author concluded that conventional TACE as well as drug-eluting beads loaded with doxorubicin and yttrium-90 (^{90}Y) microspheres demonstrated a similar median survival.

Kim and Kim [5] report that ^{90}Y radioembolization has a potent anticancer effect with negligible adverse events if appropriate pretreatment evaluations, including dosimetry, calculation of lung shunt fraction and assessment of vascular anatomy, are performed. They concluded that selected populations, for whom TACE would not be effective, are candidates for ^{90}Y radioembolization.

Peng and Chen [6] report that combination therapy of TACE with radiofrequency ablation (RFA) showed better survival and recurrence-free survival than an RFA alone group. Thus, they expect the combination therapy of TACE with RFA to become a standard of care for HCC, which is treatable with RFA, in the future.

Makino et al. [7] discuss how RFA can be performed for HCCs, which have poor conspicuity on grayscale ultrasonography (US), by introducing US fusion imaging with CT/MRI.

Inoue et al. [8] show that contrast-enhanced US (CEUS) can be used to assess the efficacy of RFA for HCC, with the potential of reducing the number of CT scans required for evaluating treatment response.

Minami and Kudo [9] examine therapeutic response assessment of TACE for HCC by US, CT and MRI. The authors conclude that CT is commonly used as the standard imaging technique, but Lipiodol makes it difficult to detect

KARGER

Fax +41 61 306 12 34
E-Mail karger@karger.com
www.karger.com

0030–2414/13/0847–0001$38.00/0

Accessible online at:
www.karger.com/ocl

Masatoshi Kudo, MD, PhD
Division of Gastroenterology and Hepatology, Department of Internal Medicine
Kinki University Faculty of Medicine
377-2 Ohno-Higashi, Osakasayama, Osaka 589-8511 (Japan)
E-Mail m-kudo@med.kindai.ac.jp

the residual tumor on CT. CEUS is a useful tool for assessing the vascularity of the viable tumor in comparison with CT. Dynamic MRI is also useful in demonstrating viable tumor with high sensitivity, but low specificity. We should keep in mind that these 3 techniques have both advantages and disadvantages in response evaluation after TACE.

Tsai et al. [10] report that serum/plasma markers, functional MRI and FDG-PET have been selectively used to predict disease outcome after radiotherapy to HCC.

Wei and Zeng [11] propose that external beam radiotherapy (EBRT) be included in the National Comprehensive Cancer Network since EBRT was more effective than sorafenib for improving patient survival when tested on tumors of comparable metastatic size.

Minata et al. [12] report that evaluating vascular endothelial growth factor in HCC tissue after surgical resection has predictive value for metastatic HCC recurrence. The ability to risk stratify should improve treatment strategies after hepatectomy.

Nishida et al. [13] discuss how methylation status of *APC* sequences could be a promising marker for improving HCC management when considering the strong association between the ratio of the methylated to unmethylated *APC* sequences in serum and the presence of portal vein thrombosis.

Minata et al. [14] show that expression levels of E-cadherin in adjacent noncancerous liver after surgical resection is associated with later metastatic HCC recurrence. Analysis of E-cadherin expression should provide important information for predicting recurrence after curative resection of HCC.

Nishida and Kudo [15] report that recent whole-genome analyses and exome sequencing of tumor DNA have revealed numerous novel alterations to cancer-related genes and pathways critical for HCC development. In addition, various risk factors for HCC, such as the presence or absence of hepatitis B and hepatitis C virus, may affect the mutation profile of the corresponding cancer genome. On the other hand, genome-wide association studies have also identified important single-nucleotide polymorphisms involved in HCC development, which may allow detection of a group at high risk of HCC emergence. Such analyses will clarify how this malignancy can be treated, diagnosed and prevented more effectively.

I believe this supplement issue contains articles with high scientific value and thus will prove to be beneficial for readers of *Oncology*.

Disclosure Statement

The author declares that no conflict of interests exist.

References

1 Fujimoto K, Kato M, Kudo M, Yada N, Shiina T, Ueshima K, et al: Novel image analysis method using ultrasound elastography for noninvasive evaluation of hepatic fibrosis in patients with chronic hepatitis C. Oncology 2013;84(suppl 1):3–13.

2 Yada N, Morikawa H, Fujimoto K, Kato M, Kawada N, Kudo M: Assessment of liver fibrosis with real-time tissue elastography in chronic viral hepatitis. Oncology 2013;84 (suppl 1):14–20.

3 Kudo M, Matsui O, Sakamoto M, Kitao A, Kim T, Ariizumi S, et al: Role of gadolinium-ethoxybenzyl-diethylenetriamine pentaacetic acid-enhanced magnetic resonance imaging in the management of hepatocellular carcinoma: consensus at the symposium of the 48th Annual Meeting of the Liver Cancer Study Group of Japan. Oncology 2013;84 (suppl 1):21–27.

4 Takayasu K: Transcatheter arterial chemoembolization for unresectable hepatocellular carcinoma: recent progression and perspective. Oncology 2013;84(suppl 1):28–33.

5 Kim YH, Kim DY: Yttrium-90 radioembolization for hepatocellular carcinoma: what we know and what we need to know. Oncology 2013;84(suppl 1):34–39.

6 Peng ZW, Chen MS: Transcatheter arterial chemoembolization combined with radiofrequency ablation for the treatment of hepatocellular carcinoma. Oncology 2013;84 (suppl 1):40–43.

7 Makino Y, Imai Y, Ohama H, Igura T, Kogita S, Sawai Y, et al: Ultrasonography fusion imaging system increases the chance of radiofrequency ablation for hepatocellular carcinoma with poor conspicuity on conventional ultrasonography. Oncology 2013;84(suppl 1):44–50.

8 Inoue T, Kudo M, Hatanaka K, Arizumi T, Takita M, Kitai S, et al: Usefulness of contrast-enhanced ultrasonography to evaluate the post-treatment responses of radiofrequency ablation for hepatocellular carcinoma: comparison with dynamic CT. Oncology 2013;84(suppl 1):51–57.

9 Minami Y, Kudo M: Therapeutic response assessment of transcatheter arterial chemoembolization for hepatocellular carcinoma: ultrasonography, CT and MR imaging. Oncology 2013;84(suppl 1):58–63.

10 Tsai CL, Koong AC, Hsu FM, Graber M, Chen IS, Cheng JCH: Biomarker studies on radiotherapy to hepatocellular carcinoma. Oncology 2013;84(suppl 1):64–68.

11 Wei J, Zeng ZC: Is it time to adopt external beam radiotherapy in the NCCN guidelines as a therapeutic strategy for intermediate/advanced hepatocellular carcinoma? Oncology 2013;84(suppl 1):69–74.

12 Minata M, Harada KH, Kudo M, Ikai I, Nishida N: The prognostic value of vascular endothelial growth factor in hepatocellular carcinoma for predicting metastasis after curative resection. Oncology 2013;84(suppl 1):75–81.

13 Nishida N, Arizumi T, Takita M, Nagai T, Kitai S, Yada N, et al: Quantification of tumor DNA in serum and vascular invasion of human hepatocellular carcinoma. Oncology 2013;84(suppl 1):82–87.

14 Minata M, Kudo M, Harada KH, Ikai I, Nishida N: Expression of E-cadherin and vascular endothelial growth factor in noncancerous liver is associated with recurrence of hepatocellular carcinoma after curative resection. Oncology 2013;84(suppl 1):86–90.

15 Nishida N, Kudo M: Recent advancements in comprehensive genetic analyses for human hepatocellular carcinoma. Oncology 2013; 84(suppl 1):91–95.

Oncology

Oncology 2013;84(suppl 1):3–12
DOI: 10.1159/000345883

Published online: February 20, 2013

Novel Image Analysis Method Using Ultrasound Elastography for Noninvasive Evaluation of Hepatic Fibrosis in Patients with Chronic Hepatitis C

Kenji Fujimoto[a, b] Michio Kato[b] Masatoshi Kudo[c] Norihisa Yada[c] Tsuyoshi Shiina[d] Kazuomi Ueshima[c] Yukinori Yamada[e] Tetsushi Ishida[f] Masayoshi Azuma[f] Masaru Yamasaki[g] Keiji Yamamoto[b] Norio Hayashi[h] Tetsuo Takehara[i]

[a]Division of Clinical Research and [b]Department of Internal Medicine, National Hospital Organization Minamiwakayama Medical Center, Tanabe, [c]Department of Gastroenterology and Hepatology, Kinki University School of Medicine, Osakasayama, [d]Human Health Sciences, Graduate School of Medicine, Kyoto University, Kyoto, Departments of [e]Gastroenterology and Hepatology, [f]Internal Medicine and [g]Clinical Laboratory, Kaizuka City Hospital, Kaizuka, [h]Department of Gastroenterology and Hepatology, Japan Labour Health and Welfare Organization, Kansai Rousai Hospital, Amagasaki, and [i]Department of Gastroenterology and Hepatology, Osaka University Graduate School of Medicine, Suita, Japan

Key Words
Real-time tissue elastography · Chronic hepatitis · Ultrasound elastography · Liver fibrosis

Abstract
It has been established that the long-term infection of chronic hepatitis C leads to the increased risk of hepatic fibrosis and hepatocellular carcinoma. Currently, histological diagnosis by invasive and painful liver biopsy is the gold standard for evaluating the hepatic fibrosis stage. Because of a side effect or patient inability to cope with the pain, it is difficult to assess the fibrosis stage frequently using liver biopsy. Recently, instead of liver biopsy, many articles have been published showing the usefulness of ultrasound elastography to evaluate the stage of hepatic fibrosis. We also reported the usefulness of real-time tissue elastography (RTE) for liver fibrosis staging in 2007. However, in our previous report, fibrosis classification was performed manually and the number of patients involved was also small. In the current study, the fibrosis staging is performed automatically using software by characterizing the elastography images. We have also increased the number of patients from 64 to 310. Thus, the aim of this study is to increase objectivity by using a newly developed automatic analysis method. We obtain the Liver Fibrosis Index (LFI), which is calculated from image features of RTE images, using multiple regression analysis performed on clinical data of 310 cases as the training data set. The correlation coefficient obtained between the LFI and the stage of hepatic fibrosis was $r = 0.68$, and significant differences exist between all stages of fibrosis ($p < 0.001$). Our new method seems promising since it has the ability to diagnose fibrosis even in the presence of inflammation.

Introduction

Approximately 700,000 people worldwide are estimated to die annually of hepatocellular carcinoma (HCC), which is the third highest cause of cancer death [1, 2]. HCC often develops in the presence of hepatic fibrosis from long-term infection of chronic hepatitis B and C. It has been reported that the risk of HCC increases as the stage of liver fibrosis progresses [3]. It has been shown that fibrosis treatment using interferon reduces hepatic

KARGER

Fax +41 61 306 12 34
E-Mail karger@karger.com
www.karger.com

0030–2414/13/0847–0003$38.00/0

Accessible online at:
www.karger.com/ocl

Masatoshi Kudo, MD, PhD
Division of Gastroenterology and Hepatology, Department of Internal Medicine
Kinki University Faculty of Medicine
377-2 Ohno-Higashi, Osakasayama, Osaka 589-8511 (Japan)
E-Mail m-kudo@med.kindai.ac.jp

Abbreviations used in this paper

MEAN	Mean of relative strain value within the ROI
SD	Standard deviation of relative strain value within the ROI
%AREA	Area of low strain (blue) within the ROI
COMP	Complexity of low strain (blue) area within the ROI = (perimeter)^2/area
SKEW	Skewness – asymmetry of the histogram
KURT	Kurtosis – peakedness of the histogram
ENT	Entropy – textural complexity
IDM	Inverse Difference Moment – textual local homogeneity
ASM	Angular Second Moment – textual homogeneity

fibrosis and also dramatically reduces the incidence of HCC [4]. Thus, it is important to evaluate the stage of hepatic fibrosis both for establishing treatment and also for monitoring its effectiveness.

Histological diagnosis using liver biopsy is very important for the evaluation of hepatic fibrosis [5–10]. However, because of its invasiveness, liver biopsy cannot be performed frequently. In addition, there is a limitation in the accuracy of liver biopsy due to sampling error [11–13]. Thus, the development of noninvasive tests that are reliable, cost-effective and easy to use is required for evaluating the stage of hepatic fibrosis. Previously, measurement of platelet counts [14] and liver fibrosis marker [15–18] were used as noninvasive tests to evaluate hepatic fibrosis, but generally the basic procedure for evaluating the stage of hepatic fibrosis is to combine the use of these tests with diagnostic imaging techniques, such as ultrasonography.

Ultrasound imaging is the most useful imaging diagnostic technique used for evaluating chronic hepatitis and/or cirrhosis. The image characteristics for evaluating hepatic fibrosis/cirrhosis are the nodular liver parenchyma, heterogeneous internal echo texture, decrease in the volume of right hepatic lobe and increase in the volume of caudate and left hepatic lobe, and the narrowing of the hepatic vein [19, 20]. However, staging of the liver fibrosis using these characteristics is less reliable since the appearance of images can be changed due to differences in ultrasonic power and/or the image settings of the equipment used. Ultrasound tissue characterization has been attempted in the literature for objective evaluation of tissue by analyzing the signals obtained from the ultrasound system, for example intensity of RF signals, extent of scattering [21, 22] and velocity of shear wave generated by a probe in the liver [23].

New methods are emerging to estimate the liver stiffness or the fibrosis, using ultrasound elastography or MRI [24]. There are many forms of elastography that are popular, namely transient elastography (Fibroscan®) [25–28], acoustic radiation forces impulse imaging (ARFI) and our own real-time tissue elastography (RTE) [29–32]. Fibroscan and ARFI measure the velocity of shear waves propagating in the tissue to measure liver stiffness, which is then correlated to fibrosis. However, in the case of Fibroscan, measured liver stiffness is correlated not only with the stage of hepatic fibrosis, but also with grade of inflammation. Therefore, the involvement of many dynamic factors independent of hepatic fibrosis affect the measurement value, such as inflammation or cholestasis. The stage of hepatic fibrosis, which is the goal of the imaging technique, should be defined as the parameter dependent only on the fibrosis of the liver, which is the true pathology to be indicated and should not include other dynamic factors.

Our RTE is different from Fibroscan and ARFI and it measures relative stiffness of the tissue in the region of interest (ROI) and displays the stiffness with color overlaid over the B-mode image in real time. Apart from liver imaging, it has many other clinical applications that have been reported in the literature, such as breast, thyroid, prostate and pancreas [33–36]. RTE image is constructed using tissue strains which are calculated from 2 consecutive frames. The phase difference of RF signals from 2 consecutive frames are calculated to obtain tissue strain and transferred to color codes. The colors in the ROI range from blue to red to show the relative hardness and softness of area inside the ROI [30, 31]. The harder areas are displayed in blue and the softer areas in red.

In our previous work using RTE for liver imaging, we established the usefulness of RTE for the evaluation of hepatic fibrosis of chronic hepatitis C patients. The reported liver elasticity scores, which were scored visually, showed significant correlation with hepatic fibrosis [37]. Our RTE, available as a native mode in an ultrasound system, can be used for evaluating patients even with ascites and severe hepatic atrophy.

Even though our previous paper showed the feasibility of using RTE, the main limitation was that the evaluation of the RTE images was performed visually. While evaluating visually, two radiologists used the increase in a blue area in the RTE image as a criteria for staging hepatic fibrosis. Blue areas of RTE images increased and became patchy as the stage of hepatic fibrosis increased. It was difficult for the radiologists to visually estimate hepatic fibrosis with RTE images since the scoring of fibrosis also depended on the individual examiner's image perspective. In addition, in our previous report, we did not perform any investigation about the relationship between the grade of inflammation and the RTE image. Thus, the aims of this study are: (1) to present a newly developed image analysis software method to obtain Liver Fibrosis Index (LFI) automatically from image features of RTE images using multiple regression analysis [38–40], (2) to show the effectiveness of this software tool and (3) to establish the relationship between LFI, the stage of fibrosis and the grade of inflammation.

Patients and Methods

Patients

The protocol was created following the Declaration of Helsinki and approved by an independent ethics committee of 3 institutions. For this study, we chose 295 patients with chronic hepatitis C or cirrhosis. Fifty-five patients were excluded from the study (table 1). All these patients were anti-hepatitis C virus and hepatitis C virus RNA positive, and were diagnosed by liver biopsy between May 2005 and December 2009. The patient population included 130 males and 165 females aged between 26 and 76 years old (mean age 56 years; table 1). Fifteen healthy volunteers were also enrolled as a normal control group. We obtained written informed consent from all participants at the National Hospital Organization Minamiwakayama Medical Center, Kaizuka City Hospital and Kinki University Hospital.

Table 1. Background of patients and excluded cases

Patients (n = 295)	
Male/female	130/165
Age, years	56 ± 18
Range	26 – 76
ALT, IU/l	59.4 ± 41.1
Total bilirubin, mg/dl	0.9 ± 0.5
Albumin, g/dl	4.0 ± 1.1
Choline esterase, IU/l	270.4 ± 78.4
Total cholesterol, mg/dl	187.4 ± 33.4
Prothrombin time, %	94.2 ± 12.9
Platelet count ($\times 10^4/\mu l$)	16.2 ± 7.7
Fibrosis stage, F0/F1/F2/F3/F4	84/97/65/48
Histological activity, A0/A1/A2/A3	29/90/146/30
Excluded cases (n = 55)	
Poor penetration (n = 20)	
Fatty layer ≥5 mm and muscular layer ≥10 mm	9
Fatty layer ≥5 mm and muscular layer <10 mm	3
Fatty layer <5 mm and muscular layer ≥10 mm	5
Fatty layer <5 mm and muscular layer <10 mm	3
Unstable technique (n = 35)	
Slipping section by body movement	10
Slipping horizontally by cardiac movement	13
Poor cardiac movement	3
Artifact by multiple reflection	9

Liver Histology

Liver biopsy was performed twice using 18G automatic cutting biopsy needles (Adjustable Temno Biopsy System; Cardinal Health, Waukegan, Ill., USA) under local anesthesia for all study patients. Regardless of benign or malignant tumor, patients who had tumor located in the imaging plane from the right intercostal were excluded from the study. The specimen lengths were 20 mm (range 10–25 mm) and the sections were stained with hematoxylin and eosin and Masson trichrome staining. These sections were examined by 3 pathologists to stage the fibrosis and also to grade the activities. All 3 pathologists were blinded to any clinical data including the results of RTE. Hepatic fibrosis were staged from F0 to F4 according to the following scale: F0 – no fibrosis, F1 – portal fibrosis without septa, F2 – portal fibrosis with septa, F3 – numerous septa without cirrhosis and F4 – cirrhosis. Inflammatory activities were graded from A0 to A3 with the following scale: A0 – no activity, A1 – mild activity, A2 – moderate activity and A3 – severe activity.

The fifteen healthy volunteers were all male, aged between 22 and 52 years (average 31.5), BMI between 17.9 and 24.7 (average 21.0) and their blood tests, such as aspartate aminotransaminase, alanine transaminase, gamma-GTP, total cholesterol and triglyceride, were all within normal limits. All volunteers had no sign of fatty liver in ultrasonography findings, thus no liver biopsy was performed and they were staged F0.

Real-Time Tissue Elastography

HI VISION 900 (Hitachi Medical Corp., Tokyo, Japan) was used for ultrasonography and the probes used were EUP-L52 linear probes (7–3 MHz). We used linear array probes for this study over convex array probes because linear probes have many advantages when internal compression and relaxation induced by the cardiac motion is utilized for obtaining RTE images of the liver. We utilized internal compression and relaxation induced by the cardiac motion instead of manual compression because this is more consistent and reliable. Even though the field of view of a linear array probe is small, the direction of displacement induced by cardiac movement can be set to the surface of the probe, thus making it suitable for RTE analysis. Also, at smaller depth the field of view of a linear probe is much larger than that of convex probes, thus making it more suitable for an RTE image.

After obtaining B-mode images, the ultrasound mode was switched to RTE and scanned from the right intercostal space to observe the right hepatic lobe. RTE images were obtained by holding the probe still at the position where displacement by the cardiac motion in B-mode was in the axial direction. The optimum intercostal space was the position where liver parenchyma was imaged in the deepest area. When the liver was not contracted, RTE images were easily obtained by scanning through the intercostal space of anterior to middle axillary lines. Because the RTE image is formed from the strain values computed from the axial displacement, the position where liver parenchyma moves in a lateral direction due to cardiac motion was not suitable for this study.

The ROI for RTE was set inside liver parenchyma. Regions with large vessels or regions having shadows from ribs were avoided to reduce the artifacts arising from the anechoic region. The tops of the ROI were positioned at a depth of more than 1 cm from the surface of the liver to avoid multiple reflections arising from the surface of the liver.

RTE was performed using a freehand technique, with the linear probe placed at the appropriate position with the patient holding their breath. As mentioned in the previous paragraph, no manual compression/relaxation was applied. The compression/

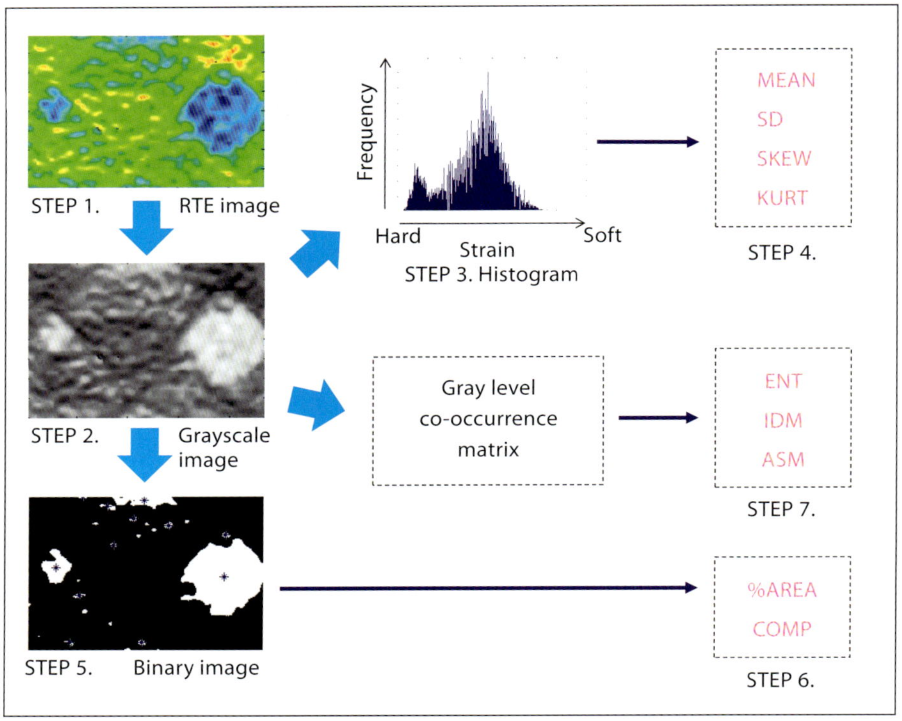

Fig. 1. Flow of calculations.

relaxation of the liver induced by the cardiac motion is easily detected to compute strain images. The ultrasound system parameters such as depth, ROI and gain were set for optimum RTE image quality. RTE images obtained by the lateral movements of the heart were avoided. One to two RTE images are displayed in 1 heartbeat, and the best RTE image was selected for final analysis. In total 3–5 RTE images obtained from different heart cycles without lateral motion were selected. The average of these 3–5 images for each patient was then used in regression analysis.

We extracted the following 9 image features to quantify the patchy pattern of the RTE images. More details about these features can also be found in the literature [41].

All 9 parameters have been found in the literature to be very useful for characterizing the imaging pattern in many different applications, e.g. satellite imaging, geothermal imaging and machine visions [42]. For liver fibrosis staging using RTE images, we employ these features for characterizing the image and correlating them with fibrosis staging. Analysis of RTE image features were performed with the prototype analysis software shown in figure 1. This software converts the selected analysis area of the RTE image (STEP 1) into a 256-step grayscale image (STEP 2), plots the strain histogram (STEP 3), and calculates the mean of relative strain (MEAN), standard deviation of relative strain (SD), skewness of strain histogram (SKEW) and kurtosis of strain histogram (KURT; STEP 4). Moreover, it binarizes the RTE image into black and white regions: white as low strain (blue) regions and black as all other regions (STEP 5). To characterize the low strain (blue) regions of the binary image, it calculates the ratio of low strain regions within the selected analysis area (%AREA), and the complexity of the low strain region (COMP; STEP 6). Furthermore, it also calculates entropy (ENT), inverse difference moment (IDM), and angular second moment (ASM) to evaluate the texture of the RTE image (STEP 7). Multiple regression analysis was then performed to improve the diagnostic accuracy using all these 9 image features instead of diagnosing with individual image features.

The LFI was estimated using these 9 image features as independent variables and the hepatic fibrosis stage as a dependent variable, as shown in the following multiple regression equation:

$$\begin{aligned} \text{LFI} = \\ &-0.009 \times \text{MEAN} - 0.005 \times \text{SD} + 0.023 \times \text{\%AREA} \\ &+ 0.025 \times \text{COMP} + 0.775 \times \text{SKEW} - 0.281 \times \text{KURT} \\ &+ 2.083 \times \text{ENT} + 3.042 \times \text{IDM} + 39.979 \times \text{ASM} - 5.542. \end{aligned}$$

Multiple regression analysis was also performed to estimate the Liver Activity Index (LAI) using 9 image features as independent variables and grade of inflammatory activity as a dependent variable. LFI and LAI were calculated for all patients and compared with the stage of hepatic fibrosis and grade of inflammatory activity. Then, to eliminate the inflammatory activity from hepatic fibrosis, LAI and grade of inflammatory activity were compared for each stage of hepatic fibrosis. Receiver operating characteristic (ROC) analysis was performed for LFI to obtain a cutoff value for the identification of F0–1/F2–4 and F0–3/F4, and also to calculate sensitivity, specificity, accuracy and area under ROC (AUROC).

Statistical Analysis

All of the statistical analysis, such as multiple regression analysis and ROC analysis were carried out using the JMP statistical discovery software, version 8.0 (SAS Institute Inc., Cary, N.C., USA) for windows.

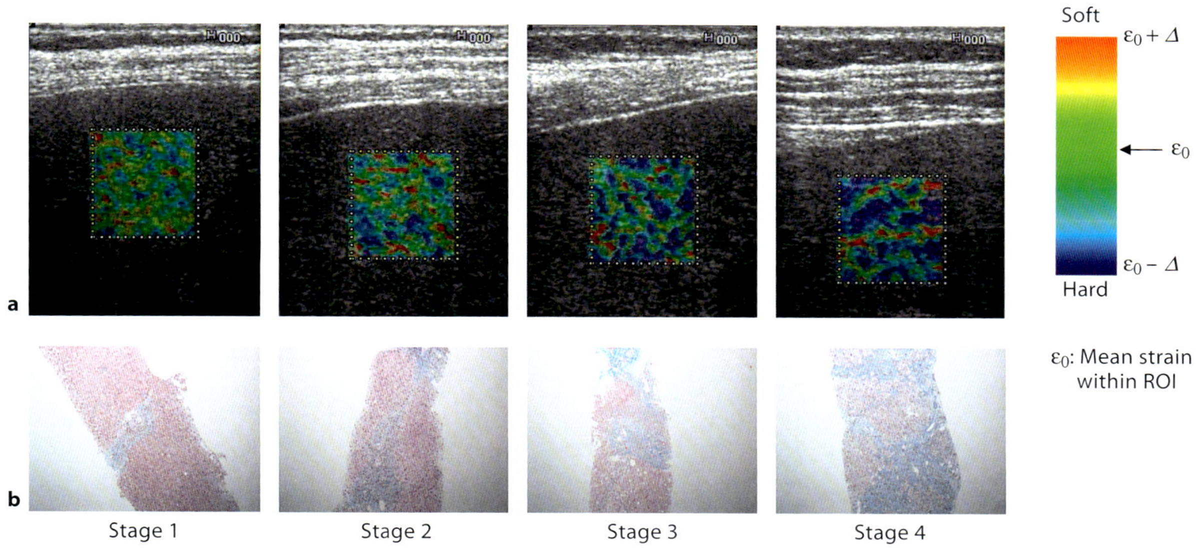

Fig. 2. RTE images (**a**) and pathological images, Masson trichrome stain, ×100 (**b**).

Results

Patients

We performed liver elastography in 365 patients (including 15 healthy volunteers) between April 2005 and November 2009. We excluded 55 patients from our study because more than 3 stable RTE images could not be acquired for these patients. Most of the reasons of exclusion were related to RTE skill of the clinicians, which improved significantly with more experience. Table 1 shows the characteristics of the 295 patients (excluding 15 healthy volunteers out of 310 patients). The indicated stages of hepatic fibrosis in the study patients were: F0 in 1 subject, F1 in 84 subjects, F2 in 97 subjects, F3 in 65 subjects and F4 in 48 subjects. The stage of hepatic fibrosis in all healthy volunteers was F0. Typical RTE images and pathological images for each fibrosis stage are shown in figure 2.

Correlation between Features and Stage

In the present study, as described previously, we extracted 9 image features. Correlation coefficients between 9 image features, such as MEAN, SD, %AREA, COMP, SKEW, KURT, ENT, IDM and ASM and stage of hepatic fibrosis were –0.63, 0.53, 0.65, 0.58, 0.59, 0.02, –0.22, 0.34 and 0.21, respectively. Thus, 5 of 9 image features, i.e. MEAN, SD, %AREA, COMP and SKEW, highly correlated with the stage of hepatic fibrosis (fig. 3).

Accuracy of Staging Fibrosis by LFI

Figure 4 shows the relationship between hepatic fibrosis stages and LFI calculated from 9 image features using multiple regression analysis. LFI highly correlates with the fibrosis stages ($r = 0.68$ with $p < 0.001$), and significant differences exist between all different stages. Figure 5 shows the ROC analysis. When the cutoff value of LFI was set to 1.92, the AUROC of LFI for F0–1 versus F2–4 was 0.82, and sensitivity, specificity and accuracy were 78.6, 78.0 and 78.4%, respectively. For F0–3 versus F4, when the cutoff value was 2.56, the AUROC was 0.87, and sensitivity, specificity and accuracy were 79.2, 80.5 and 80.3%, respectively (fig. 5). In this study, LFI clearly differentiates either F0–1 and F2–4 or F0–3 and F4.

Effect of Inflammation

Figure 6 shows the comparison between grades and the 9 image features for evaluating the effect of inflammation on RTE image. None of the 9 image features have a correlation with grades, and LAI, which was calculated by multiple regression analysis similar to LFI, also did not correlate with grades ($r = 0.30$; fig. 6j).

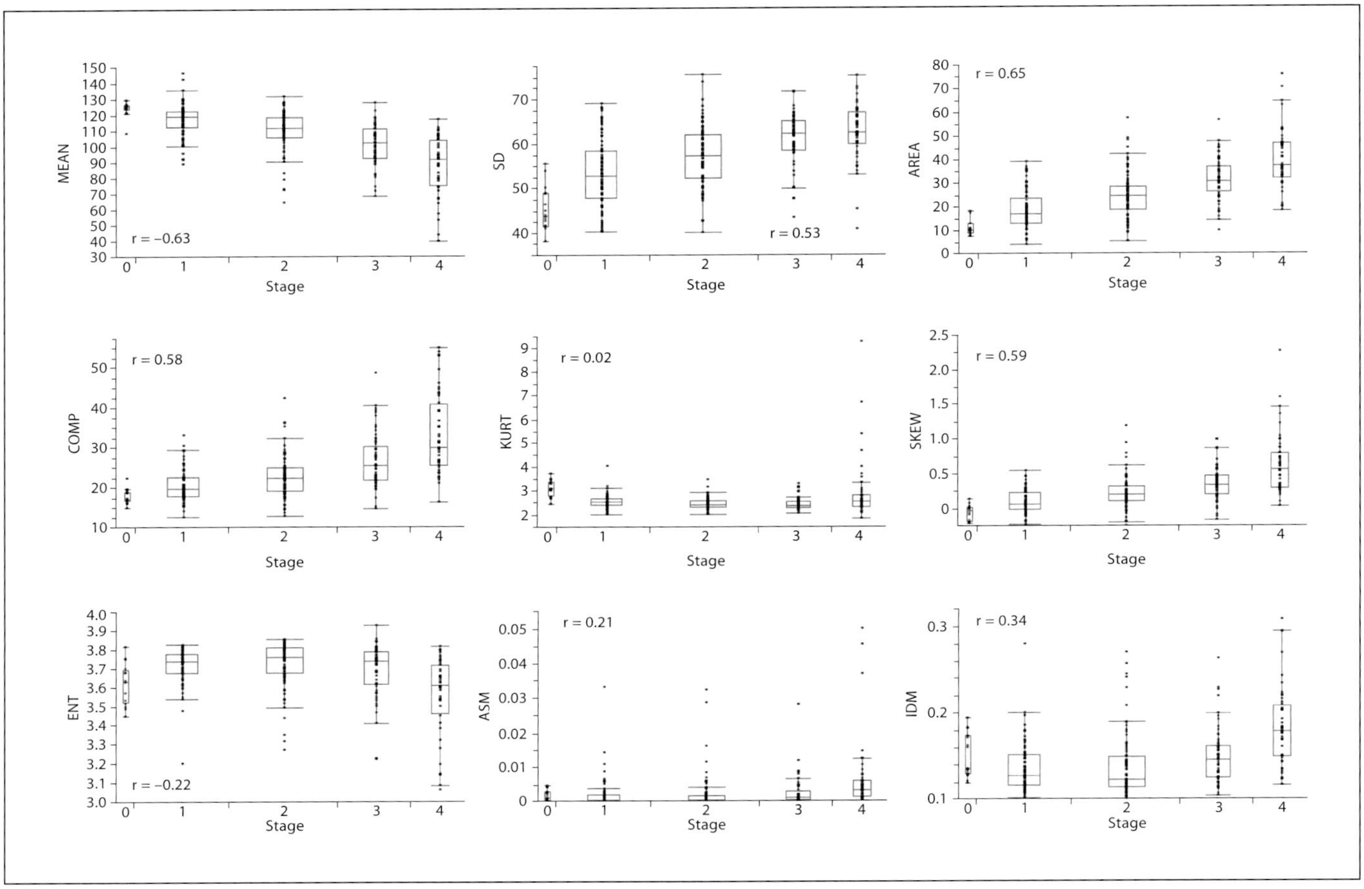

Color version available online

Fig. 3. Comparisons of stage of hepatic fibrosis and image features.

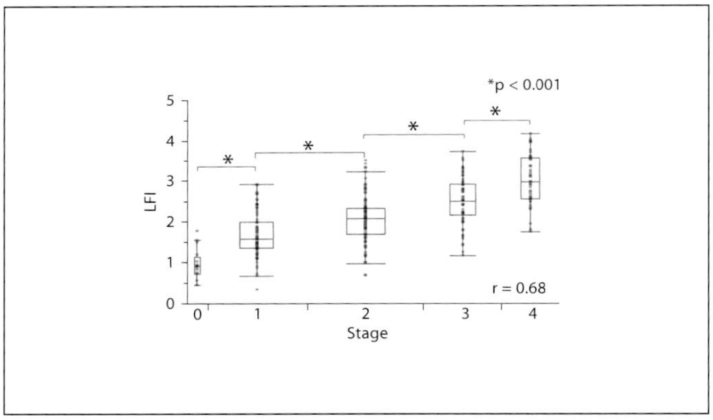

Color version available online

Fig. 4. Comparison of stage of hepatic fibrosis and LFI.

Discussion

Results of Estimation

To improve the accuracy of estimation of hepatic fibrosis and to make it automatic, we performed multiple regression analysis using 9 image features and obtained the estimated LFI. This index highly correlated with the stage of hepatic fibrosis (r = 0.68, $p < 0.001$) and significant differences were also observed between each stage. Furthermore, ROC analysis indicated that LFI has a high ability to differentiate each stage.

All 9 image features we used are independent and do not include confounding factors. Out of the 9 image features we analyzed, 5 (%AREA, MEAN, SD, COMP and SKEW) had a high correlation with the stages of hepatic fibrosis. This strong correlation, we believe, is mainly due to following reasons:

- AREA: hard area increases as a hepatic fibrosis progresses.

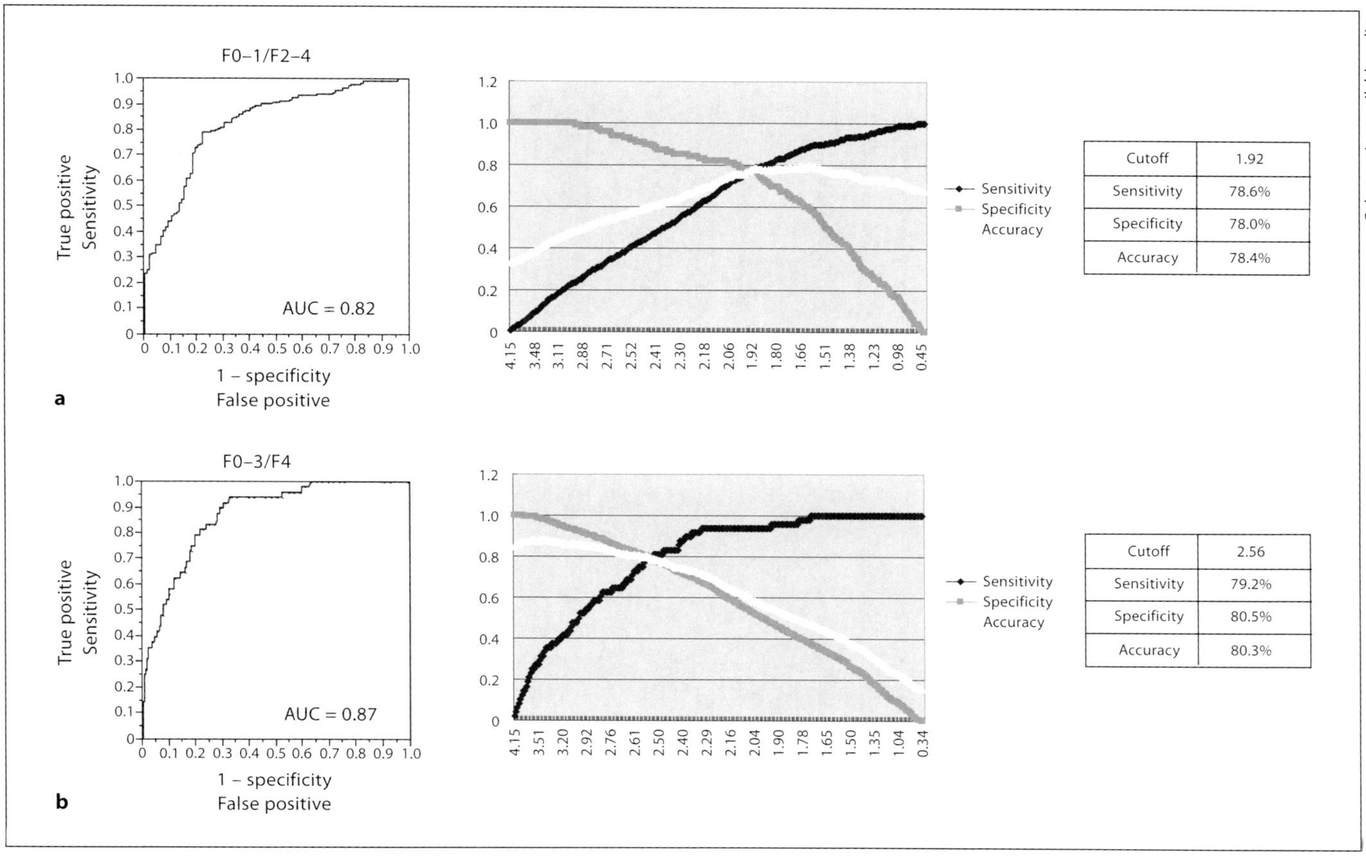

Color version available online

Fig. 5. ROC analysis differentiating F2–4 from F0–1 (**a**) and F4 from F0–3 (**b**).

- MEAN: liver parenchyma becomes stiffer as hepatic fibrosis progresses.
- SD: stiffness of liver parenchyma becomes heterogeneous as hepatic fibrosis progresses.
- COMP: figure of hard area becomes more complex as hepatic fibrosis progresses.
- SKEW: histogram skew towards the lower value of strain (harder) as hepatic fibrosis progresses.

Histopathological tissue evaluation using liver biopsy has been the gold standard for evaluation of hepatic fibrosis. However, this procedure is invasive, painful and could cause complications, such as hemorrhage, due to which many patients hesitate over the procedure. In addition, if the platelet count is low, partial thromboplastin time is greater than 3 s, the liver presents with a tumor and there is presence of ascites, then liver biopsy is also difficult to perform. This liver biopsy is also an economic burden due to the hospitalization required after the procedure. Currently, in such patients where a liver biopsy cannot be performed it is substituted with blood tests, which have significantly lower accuracy. Thus, our LFI based on RTE images, which is painless, cost-effective and can be performed in the presence of any of the above conditions can be a good addition to the clinicians tools for the noninvasive evaluation of liver fibrosis.

Effect of Inflammation

We did not find any correlation between any of the 9 features we used and inflammation grades. The RTE image, we believe, thus reflects the hepatic fibrosis and does not reflect the inflammatory factors such as intracellular pressure and change in blood flow due to inflammation. In addition, the spatial resolution of RTE images is 0.5–2 mm [43], which can completely capture the regenerating nodules in liver cirrhosis, which are 3–10 mm in size [44]. Thus, we can conclude that the LFI we have developed is not influenced by inflammation and it depends mainly upon liver fibrosis. Compared to RTE, other shear wave elastogra-

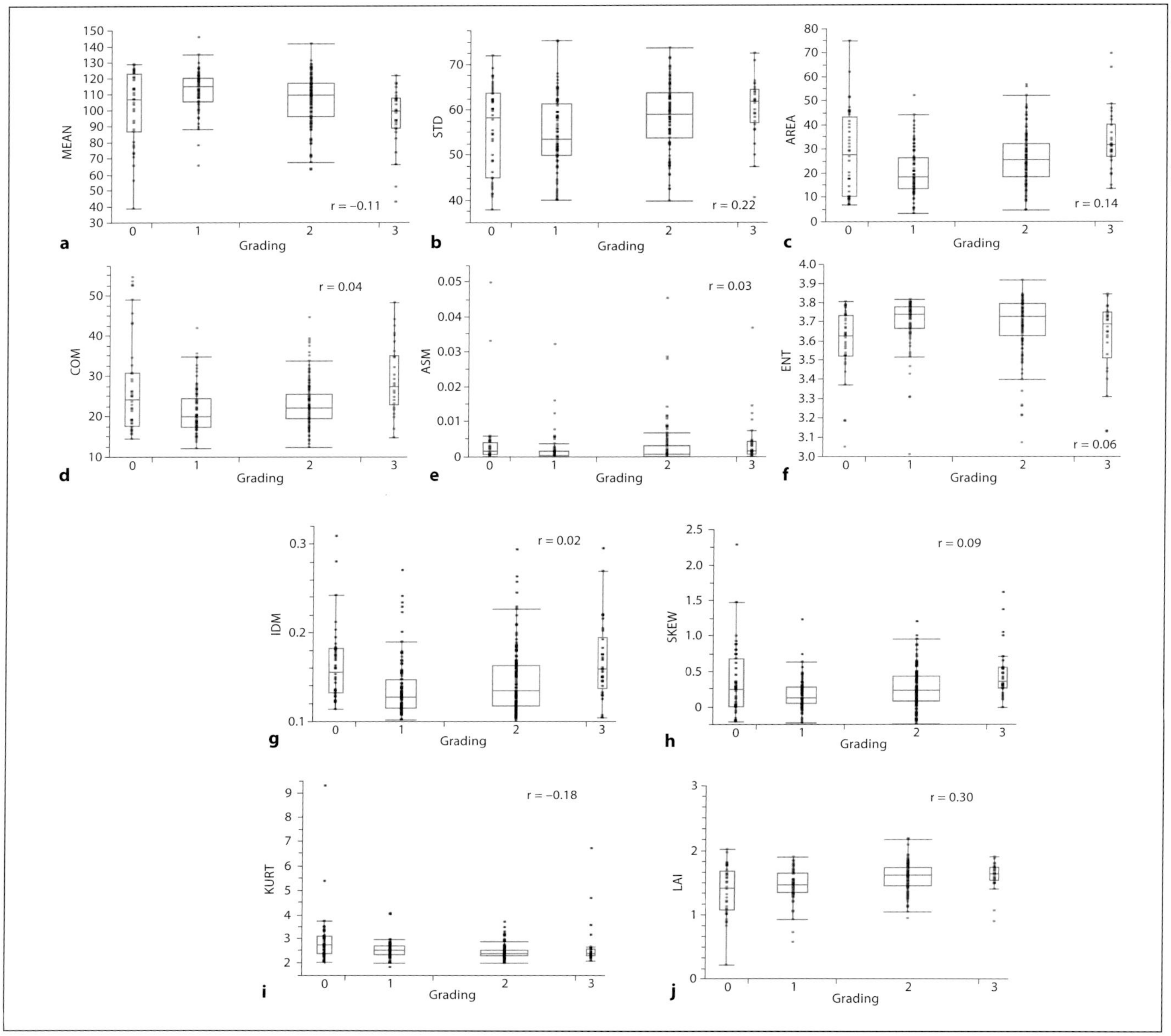

Color version available online

Fig. 6. a–j Comparison of grade and image features.

phy-based techniques, such as Fibroscan and ARFI, have been reported showing strong correlation with inflammation [45–47]. This correlation could be mainly because shear wave elastography adopts the principle of measuring the velocity of shear wave. Inflammatory factors such as intracellular pressure and condition of blood flow may change the velocity of shear waves, thus resulting in bias in the estimate.

Acquisition of RTE

We utilized compression/relaxation induced by the cardiac motion to obtain our RTE images for liver index computation. This helped to simplify RTE image acquisition and made it easier for clinicians to acquire RTE images. However, for some patients with weak pulsation and/or who are obese, it was difficult to perform liver elastography accurately. Training of clinicians was needed to avoid artifacts related to obesity, to set the ROI not to include vessels and to adjust the position of the probe to image the liver where compression/relaxation was homogeneous and axial to the probe. RTE data were collected in 3 hospitals and 2 experts performed liver elastography. Image features were extracted from multiple RTE images and the average value from the acquired RTE images were used for our analysis.

Patient Selection Bias

In our study we did not include patients who had difficulty holding their breath or for whom it was difficult to image the liver through the intercostal spaces due to overlying bowel gases. Moreover, we excluded 55 cases with difficulty in analysis, the reasons for which are shown in table 1. The acquisition rate was 84.9% (310/365), which is still quite impressive in spite of these exclusions. Most of the exclusions happened at the beginning of the study. As the clinician gained experience, the failure rate reduced significantly and the success rate increased up to 98.0% (98/100). This implies that with some education and training the acquisition failure rate can be decreased significantly.

Limitations

We compared the results of LFI derived from RTE images with histopathological results of liver biopsy. However, liver biopsy results themselves have bias due to sampling error and due to the histopathological image being classified not by continuous quantity but staged by the progression of hepatic fibrosis. Moreover, there are large differences in the progression of hepatic fibrosis between 4 stages of liver fibrosis [40], thus the accuracy of liver biopsy is limited. Since liver biopsy results are used as a training set for our LFI computation, we speculate that there is also some bias in our estimate of liver fibrosis. A new index is needed as training data to derive a multiple regression equation to reduce the variation in results.

As a future subject for increasing the accuracy of the LFI, fibrosis staging by two or more pathologists is due to be judged using the block specimen by a surgical resection. Thereby, since the variation in a pathology result can be decreased, we think that better equation estimates of LFI can be derived.

Prospects of RTE

Our results of liver fibrosis staging are very impressive. It is automatic, consistent and agrees very well with current liver biopsy results. Thus, in the near future, we expect that the RTE could be used as a first-choice imaging tool for fibrosis screening. If considered suspicious, then liver biopsy can be performed for further confirmation. In addition, RTE imaging could be the only choice available along with blood tests for patients in whom liver biopsy cannot be performed. RTE can also be used for monitoring the progress or resolution of fibrosis in patients treated with interferon. It can also be used to monitor the progress in fibrosis in patients where interferon treatment was not done. RTE imaging is easy to use, cost-effective and, moreover, painless. It is readily available with the ultrasound machine as an additional mode making the technique easily available and easy to use when liver screening is being done to monitor cirrhosis and rule out HCC. It can also be used in patients with hepatitis other than viral, such as nonalcoholic steatohepatitis, etc.

Conclusion

LFI computed from RTE images highly correlates with stages of hepatic fibrosis and accurately reflects the underlying hepatic fibrosis, even with the presence of inflammation. Thus, it can be used for screening, monitoring and at times diagnosis of hepatic fibrosis. We believe our results and our techniques are superior to other techniques such as transient elastography. In the near future we plan to conduct more extensive clinical studies both for substantiating our results as well as to prove the clinical utility of RTE imaging for liver fibrosis staging.

Acknowledgments

We would like to thank Akiko Tonomura, Tsuyoshi Mitake, Mitsuru Motoki, Tomoko Furuta, MD, Chie Tatsumi, MD, Shigeo Wada, MD and Masahide Oshita, MD, for valuable contributions to this study.

Disclosure Statement

The authors declare that no conflicts of interest exist.

References

1 WHO International Agency for Research on Cancer: World Cancer Report 2008. Section 1 – global cancer control, chapter 1.3: worldwide cancer burden. http://www.iarc.fr/en/publications/pdfs-online/wcr/2008/index.php.

2 WHO International Agency for Research on Cancer: World Cancer Report 2008. Section 2 – etiology of cancer, chapter 2.5: chronic Infections.

3 Yoshida H, Shiratori Y, Moriyama M, et al: Interferon therapy reduces the risk for hepatocellular carcinoma: national surveillance program of cirrhotic and noncirrhotic patients with chronic hepatitis C in Japan. Ann Intern Med 1999;131:174–181.
4 Shiratori Y, Imazeki F, Moriyama M, et al: Histologic improvement of fibrosis in patients with hepatitis C who have sustained response to interferon therapy. Ann Intern Med 2000;132:517–524.
5 Desmet VJ, Gerber M, Hoofnagle JH, et al: Classification of chronic hepatitis: diagnosis, grading and staging. Hepatology 1994; 19:1513–1520.
6 Ichida F, Tsuji T, Omata M, et al: Classification report: new inuyama classification for histological assessment of chronic hepatitis. Internat Hepatol Comm 1996;6:112–119.
7 Ishak K, Baptista A, Bianchi L, et al: Histological grading and staging of chronic hepatitis. J Hepatol 1995;22:696.
8 Bataller R, Brenner DA: Liver fibrosis. J Clin Invest 2005;115:209–218.
9 Pinzani M, Rombouts K, Colagrande S: Fibrosis in chronic liver diseases: diagnosis and management. J Hepatol 2005;42:S22–S26.
10 Dienstag JL: The role of liver biopsy in chronic hepatitis C. Hepatology 2002;36: S152–S160.
11 Gebo KA, Herlong HF, Torbenson MS, et al: Role of liver biopsy in management of chronic hepatitis C: a systemic review. Hepatology 2002;36:161–172.
12 Regev A, Berho M, Jeffers LJ, Milikowski C, et al: Sampling error and intraobserver variation in liver biopsy in patients with chronic HCV infection. Am J Gastroenterol 2002;97: 2614–2618.
13 Bedossa P, Dargère D, Paradis V: Sampling variability of liver fibrosis in chronic hepatitis C. Hepatology 2003;38:1449–1457.
14 Omata M: A strategy of the treatment for the viral hepatitis (in Japanese). J Jpn Soc Int Med 2004;93:269–276.
15 Manning DS, Afdhai NH: Diagnosis and quantitation of fibrosis. Gastroenterology, 2008;134:1670–1681.
16 Wai CT, Greenson JK, Fontana RJ, et al: A simple noninvasive index can predict both significant fibrosis and cirrhosis in patients with chronic hepatitis C. Hepatology 2003; 38:518–526.
17 Imbert-Bismut F, Ratziu, Pieroni L, Charlotte F, et al: Biochemical markers of liver fibrosis in patients with hepatitis C virus infection: a prospective study. Lancet 2001;357: 1069–1075.
18 Forns X, Ampurdanes S, Llovet JM, et al: Indentification of chronic hepatitis C patients without hepatic fibrosis by a simple predictive model. Hepatology 2001;36:986–992.
19 Freeman MP, Vick CW, Taylor KJ, et al: Regenerating nodules in cirrhosis: sonographic appearance with anatomic correlation. AJR Am J Roentgenol 1986;146:533–536.
20 Ishikawa H, Ono M, Goto M, et al: Ultrasonographic findings in patients with liver cirrhosis; relationships between parenchymal, superficial echo patterns, and histological findings (in Japanese). Jpn J Med Ultrason 1990;17:522–529.
21 Fujimoto K, Yamamoto Y, Waki H, et al: Tissue characterization using integrated backscatter in viral chronic liver disease. J Ultrasound Med 1999;18(suppl):472.
22 Kumada T, Toyoda H, Ogawa S, et al: Quantification of fibrosis in hepatitis C using statistics analysis tool of ultrasonics (2nd report). Jpn J Med Ultrasonics 2007;34:S641.
23 Ziol M, Handra-Luca A, Kettaneh A, et al: Noninvasive assessment of liver fibrosis by measurement of stiffness in patients with chronic hepatitis C. Hepatology 2005;41:48–54.
24 Joo I, Choi BI: New Paradigm for management of hepatocellular carcinoma by imaging. Liver Cancer 2012;1:94–109.
25 Sandrin L, Fourquet B, Hasquenoph JM, et al: Transient elastography: a new noninvasive method for assessment of hepatic fibrosis. Ultrasound Med Biol 2003;29:1705–1713.
26 Foucher J, Chanteloup E, Vergniol J, et al: Diagnosis of cirrhosis by transient elastography (FibroScan): a prospective study. Gut 2006;55:403–408.
27 Fraquelli M, Rigamonti C, Casazza G, et al: Reproducibility of transient elastography in the evaluation of liver fibrosis in patients with chronic liver disease. Gut 2007;56:968–973.
28 Kim DY, Kim SU, Park JY, Ahn SH, Song KJ, Han KH: FibroScan based risk estimation of HBV-related HCC occurrence: development and validation of a predictive model. Liver Cancer 2012;1:123.
29 Friedrich-Rust M, Wunder K, Kriener S, et al: Liver fibrosis in viral hepatitis: noninvasive assessment with acoustic radiation force impulse imaging versus transient elastography. Radiology 2009;252:595–604.
30 Shiina T, Nitta N, Ueno E, et al: Real time tissue elasticity imaging using the combined autocorrelation method. J Med Ultrasonics 1999;26:57–66.
31 Shiina T, Nitta N, Ueno E, et al: Real time tissue elasticity imaging using the combined autocorrelation method. J Med Ultrasonics 2002;29:119–128.
32 Joo I, Choi BI: New paradigm for management of hepatocellular carcinoma by imaging. Liver Cancer 2012;1:94–109.
33 Itoh A, Ueno E, Tohno E, et al: Breast disease: clinical application of US elastography for diagnosis. Radiology 2006;239:341–350.
34 Fukunari N: More accurate and sensitive diagnosis for thyroid tumors with elastography – detection and differential diagnosis of thyroid cancers. MEDIX Suppl. 2007. http://www.hitachi-medical.co.jp/tech/medix/pdf/supple/sup_05.pdf.
35 Tsutsumi M, Miyagawa T, Matsumura T, et al: Real-time balloon inflation elastography for prostate cancer detection and initial evaluation of clinic pathologic analysis, AJR Am J Roentgenol 2010;194:W471–W476.
36 Hirooka Y, Itoh A, Kawashima H, et al: Diagnosis of pancreatic disorders using contrast-enhanced endoscopic ultrasonography and endoscopic elastography. Clin Gastroenterol Hepatol 2009;7:S63–S67.
37 Fujimoto K, Wada S, Oshita M, et al: Noninvasive evaluation of hepatic fibrosis in patients with chronic hepatitis C using elastography. MEDIX Suppl. 2007. http://www.hitachi-medical.co.jp/tech/medix/pdf/supple/sup_07.pdf.
38 Tatsumi C, Kudo M, Ueshima K, et al: Noninvasive evaluation of hepatic fibrosis using serum fibrotic markers, transient elastography (FibroScan), and real-time tissue elastography. Intervirology 2008;1:S27–S33.
39 Tatsumi C, Kudo M, Ueshima K, et al: Noninvasive evaluation of hepatic fibrosis for type C chronic hepatitis. Intervirology 2010; 53:76–81.
40 Fujimoto K, Kato M, Tonomura A, et al: Non-invasive evaluation method of the liver fibrosis using real-time tissue elastography – usefulness of judgment liver fibrosis stage by Liver Fibrosis Index (LF Index) (in Japanese). Kanzo 2010;51:539–541.
41 Haralick RM, Shanmugan K, Dinstein I: Textural features for image classification. IEEE Trans Syst Man Cybern 1973;3:610–621.
42 Mittal D, Kumara V, et al: Neural network based focal liver lesion diagnosis using ultrasound images. Comp Med Imaging Graphics 2011;35:315–323.
43 Matsumura T, Shiina T, Oosaka T, et al: Development of real-time tissue elastography (in Japanese). MEDIX 2004;41:30–35.
44 Hoon L, Kim Y, Lee J: Regenerative nodules in liver cirrhosis: findings at CT during arterial portography and CT hepatic arteriography with histopathologic correlation. Radiology 1999;210:451–458.
45 Arena U, Vizzutti F, Abraldes JG, et al: Reliability of transient elastography for the diagnosis of advanced fibrosis in chronic hepatitis C. Gut 2008;57:1288–1293.
46 Vispo E, Barreiro P, Del Valle J, et al: Overestimation of liver fibrosis staging using transient elastography in patients with chronic hepatitis C and significant liver inflammation. Antivir Ther 2009;14:187–193.
47 Rifai K, Cornberg J, Mederacke I, et al: Clinical feasibility of liver elastography by acoustic radiation force impulse imaging (ARFI). Dig Liver Dis 2011;43:491–497.

Oncology

Oncology 2013;84(suppl 1):13–20
DOI: 10.1159/000345884

Published online: February 20, 2013

Assessment of Liver Fibrosis with Real-Time Tissue Elastography in Chronic Viral Hepatitis

Norihisa Yada[a] Masatoshi Kudo[a] Hiroyasu Morikawa[b] Kenji Fujimoto[c, d]
Michio Kato[d] Norifumi Kawada[b]

[a]Department of Gastroenterology and Hepatology, Kinki University Faculty of Medicine, Osakasayama,
[b]Department of Hepatology, Graduate School of Medicine, Osaka City University, Osaka, and
[c]Division of Clinical Research and [d]Department of Internal Medicine, National Hospital Organization, Minamiwakayama Medical Center, Tanabe, Japan

Key Words
Real-time tissue elastography · FibroScan · Liver fibrosis · Liver stiffness

Abstract
Objective: The aim of this study was to assess prospectively the accuracy of measurement of liver fibrosis with real-time tissue elastography (RTE) in patients with chronic viral hepatitis. ***Methods:*** Two hundred and forty-five patients were prospectively enrolled. Nine image features were measured from strain images, and Liver Fibrosis Index (LFI) was calculated from these features. Fibrosis stage was diagnosed from pathological specimens obtained by ultrasound-guided biopsy. LFI and serological markers were compared with pathological diagnosis, and the diagnostic performance of RTE was compared. ***Results:*** LFI in stages F0–F1, F2, F3 and F4 was 1.58, 2.03, 2.40 and 2.86, respectively, demonstrating a stepwise increase with increasing severity of liver fibrosis ($p < 0.001$). LFI in F2 did not significantly differ from that in F3, whereas for all other combinations of stages, there were significant differences. The area under the receiver operating characteristic curve of the LFI, platelet count, aspartate/alanine aminotransferase ratio, aspartate aminotransferase-to-platelet ratio, and FibroIndex for predicting F3 stage or higher (F0–F2 vs. F3–F4) was 0.865, 0.824, 0.708, 0.789 and 0.828, respectively. ***Conclusions:*** RTE is useful for diagnosis of liver fibrosis, regardless of stage, in patients with chronic viral hepatitis.

Introduction

The assessment of liver fibrosis is an important factor in deciding on therapeutic options and for predicting the prognosis of chronic hepatitis. Biopsy is the gold standard for assessment of liver fibrosis; however, it carries risks such as bleeding and pain. Furthermore, needle biopsy of the liver has been shown to be associated with a high rate of sampling error in patients with diffuse parenchymal liver diseases. The possibility of sampling error with liver biopsy arises because the tissue obtained represents only a small portion (approx. one part in 50,000) of the entire liver mass [1–3].

Elastography is reported to be useful for diagnosis of liver fibrosis and has a variety of measurement methods [4, 5]. FibroScan, virtual-touch tissue quantification, and shear wave elastography measure the propagation speed

KARGER

Fax +41 61 306 12 34
E-Mail karger@karger.com
www.karger.com

0030–2414/13/0847–0013$38.00/0

Accessible online at:
www.karger.com/ocl

Masatoshi Kudo, MD, PhD
Division of Gastroenterology and Hepatology, Department of Internal Medicine
Kinki University Faculty of Medicine
377-2 Ohno-Higashi, Osakasayama, Osaka 589-8511 (Japan)
E-Mail m-kudo@med.kindai.ac.jp

of the shear wave [6–8]. The more severe hepatic fibrosis progresses, the faster propagation speed increases. They are said to be useful for the diagnosis of liver fibrosis, especially in advanced fibrosis cases. However, the propagation speed of the shear wave is not only affected by liver fibrosis, but also hepatic activity, jaundice and hepatic congestion [9–12]. The other method measures tissue distortion. Real-time tissue elastography (RTE) shows in real time the strain of the tissue. It has been reported that RTE is useful for evaluation of malignant tumors in the mammary gland and thyroid [13, 14].

In the present study, we investigated the performance of RTE for diagnosis of liver fibrosis. We also compared the diagnostic performance of RTE and serum markers of fibrosis.

Patients and Methods

Patients

This was a multicenter, cross-sectional study that was performed at Kinki University Hospital (Osaka, Japan), Osaka City University Hospital (Osaka, Japan) and Minamiwakayama Medical Center (Wakayama, Japan). Consecutive patients with chronic hepatitis C virus (HCV) or chronic by hepatitis B virus (HBV) infection, who underwent percutaneous ultrasound-guided liver biopsy before treatment, were enrolled. Only patients with HCV or HBV, whose disease was defined by the presence of serum anti-HCV antibody and serum HCV RNA, or the presence of serum hepatitis B surface antibody and serum HBV DNA, were included. Percutaneous ultrasound-guided liver biopsy was performed within 2 weeks before or after RTE. Clinical and laboratory data were collected at the time of liver biopsy. Patients were excluded if they consumed >20 g alcohol per day. Patients with a history of autoimmune hepatitis, primary biliary hepatitis, primary sclerosing cholangitis, hemochromatosis, α1-antitrypsin deficiency, or Wilson's disease were also excluded. The study protocol conformed to the Declaration of Helsinki and was approved by the local ethics committee. Informed consent to participate in the study was obtained from each patient.

Clinical and Laboratory Assessments

Relevant clinical data recorded were age, sex, weight, height, waist circumference and cause of chronic liver disease. Body Mass Index was calculated as weight (kg) divided by height (m) squared. Blood samples were taken after overnight fasting on the day of biopsy. Laboratory tests including platelet count, cholesterol, bilirubin, aspartate aminotransferase (AST), alanine aminotransferase (ALT), γ-glutamyl transpeptidase, bilirubin, albumin, γ-globulins, prothrombin time and international normalized ratio were assessed using automated methods. From these single variables, three ratio indexes were calculated using classical ratios: AST/ALT [15]; AST-to-platelet ratio index [APRI; AST/upper limit of normal 100/platelet count (10^4/mm^3)] [16], and FibroIndex [1.738 – 0.064 × platelet count (10^4/mm^3) + 0.005 × AST (U/l) + 0.463 × γ-globulin (g/dl)] [17].

Liver Histological Assessment

Percutaneous ultrasound-guided liver biopsy was performed on the liver right lobe with a Tru-Cut semiautomatic 18-gauge needle apparatus (Monopty; C.R. Bard, Tempe, Ariz., USA). The liver biopsy specimens were fixed in formalin, embedded in paraffin and stained with hematoxylin and eosin, Masson's trichrome or Azan stain. All biopsy specimens were examined by pathologists who were blinded to the patient characteristics. Liver fibrosis was scored by the New Inuyama classification. The stage of fibrosis was classified from F0 to F4 as follows: F0, no fibrosis; F1, fibrosis portal expansion; F2, bridging fibrosis (portal–portal or portal–central linkage); F3, bridging fibrosis with lobular distortion (disorganization), and F4, cirrhosis.

Real-Time Tissue Elastography

RTE was performed using ultrasonography (EUS-8500, HI-VISION 900 and HI-VISION Ascendus; Hitachi Aloka Medical, Tokyo, Japan) and the EUP-L52 linear probe (3–7 MHz; Hitachi Aloka Medical). Patients were examined in the spine position with the right arm in maximal abduction and were instructed to hold their breath. The examinations were performed on the right lobe of the liver through the intercostal spaces, holding firmly the transducer without applying compression on the skin. The B-mode and static image superimposed on B-mode were both visualized in real-time; therefore, the best position could be easily selected. The region of interest (ROI) of the strain image was 2.5 cm^2 and located about 1 cm below the surface of the liver. In addition, to obtain good images, scanning was performed to avoid large vessels and attenuation by lungs and ribs. RTE shows a relative strain image, thus, there should be no artifacts in the ROI of the strain image.

Nine image features were extracted from each RTE image: mean relative strain value (MEAN); standard deviation of relative strain value (SD); percentage of low strain area (percentage of blue color area – %AREA); complexity of low strain area (calculated as perimeter^2/area – COMP); skewness (SKEW); kurtosis (KURT); entropy (ENT); textural complexity, inverse difference moment (IDM), and angular second moment (ASM). For stable extracting of image features, the extraction area approximately matched or was slightly smaller than the ROI of the strain image (fig. 1). To perform a quantitative evaluation, Liver Fibrosis Index (LFI) was calculated as follows: –0.009 × MEAN – 0.005 × SD + 0.023 × %AREA + 0.025 × COMP + 0.775 × SKEW – 0.281 × KURT + 2.083 × ENT + 3.042 × IDM + 39.979 × ASM – 5.542 [18, 19]. The median LFI was calculated from 10 images.

Statistical Analysis

Descriptive statistics are shown as the mean ± SD, median or percentage, as appropriate. Comparisons between groups were determined by Wilcoxon's signed rank test and confirmed by the nonparametric Mann-Whitney U test between groups. Correlation between data was tested using the nonparametric Spearman rank correlation analysis. Differences were considered statistically significant at $p < 0.05$. Tukey's Honestly Significant Difference test was used to compare the data among each fibrosis stage of chronic hepatitis. The diagnostic performance for liver fibrosis was determined in terms of sensitivity, specificity, positive predictive value, negative predictive value, diagnostic accuracy and area under the receiver operating characteristic curve (AUROC). Analysis was performed using SPSS Statistics 20 (IBM, Armonk, N.Y., USA).

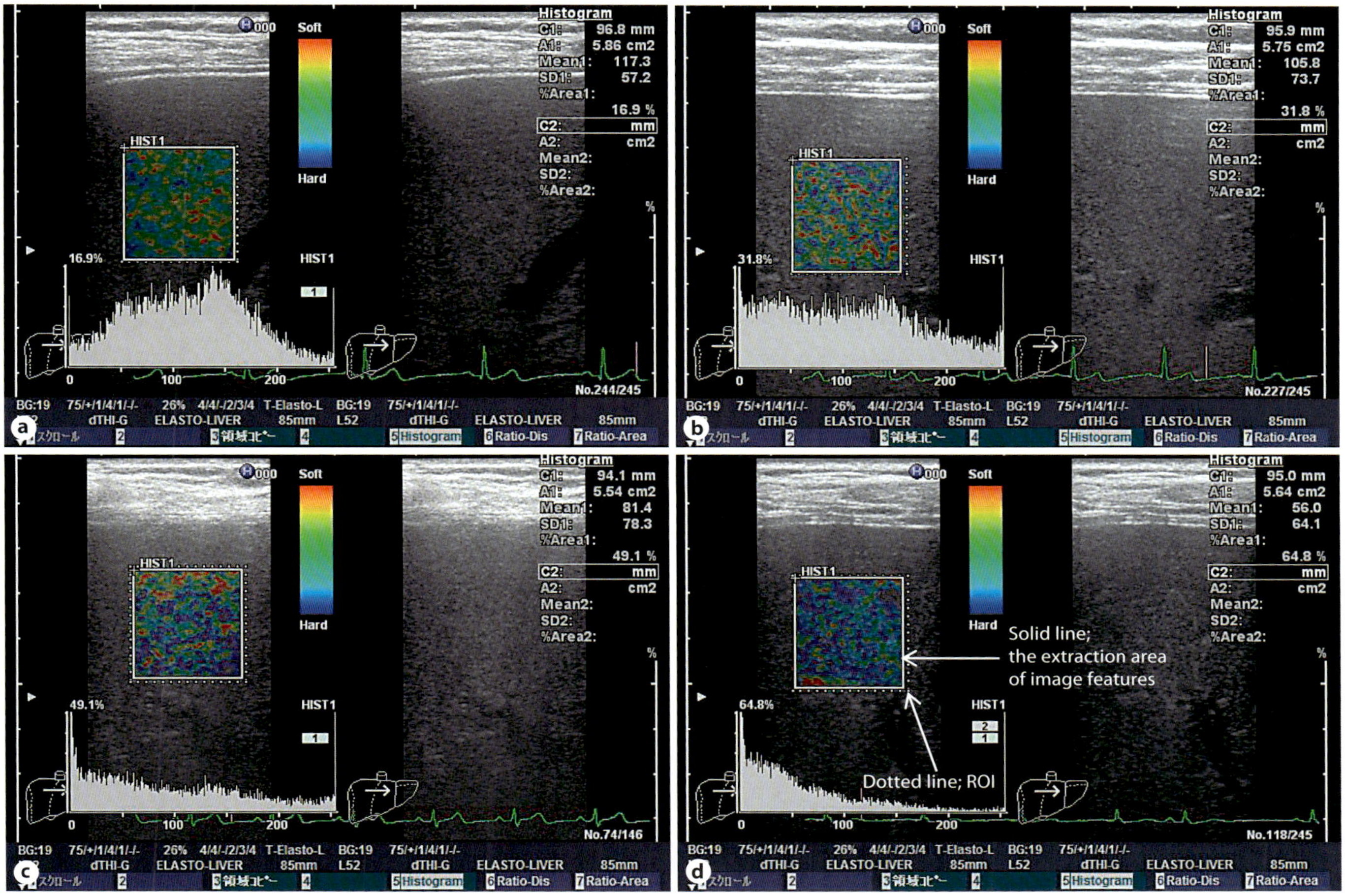

Fig. 1. RTE images in patients with chronic viral hepatitis. With fibrosis associated to progress, strain elastogram increases color variation between relatively low strain regions and generates a patched image pattern. F1 stage (**a**), F2 stage (**b**), F3 stage (**c**), F4 stage (**d**).

Results

Demographics and Baseline Features

In 4 patients, the liver biopsy specimen was too small to be used for pathological diagnosis. The remaining 245 patients, 137 (56.1%) men and 108 women (43.9%) who met the requirements were enrolled in the study. The clinical characteristics and laboratory data are shown in table 1. One hundred and eighty-nine patients (77.1%) had HCV and the other 56 (22.9%) had HBV. Four, 95, 77, 27 and 42 patients were respectively diagnosed with stage F0, F1, F2, F3 and F4 fibrosis. AST and alkaline phosphatase were significantly elevated with increasing severity of fibrosis ($p < 0.001$). Serum albumin, cholinesterase, total cholesterol, prothrombin time and platelet count were significantly decreased with increasing severity of fibrosis ($p < 0.001$).

Comparison of Serological Markers and Pathological Diagnosis

Serological fibrosis makers, platelet count, AST/ALT ratio, APRI and FibroIndex were compared with the pathological diagnosis of hepatic fibrosis. Platelet count in patients with F0–F1, F2, F3 and F4 stage fibrosis was 21.0, 15.7, 14.1 and 10.6 × $10^4/mm^3$, respectively, demonstrating a stepwise decrease with increasing severity of liver fibrosis ($p < 0.001$). AST/ALT ratio in patients with F0–F1, F2, F3 and F4 stage fibrosis was 1.09, 1.01, 1.59 and 1.33, respectively, and showed a slightly upward trend with increasing severity of liver fibrosis ($p = 0.001$). APRI in patients with F0–F1, F2, F3, and F4 stage fibrosis was 5.49, 11.37, 12.52 and 23.79, respectively, and FibroIndex in patients with F0–F1, F2, F3 and F4 stage was 1.21, 1.78, 1.82, and 2.31, respectively. Both APRI and FibroIndex

Table 1. Clinical characteristics and laboratory data of patients

Fibrosis stage	F0–F1	F2	F3	F4	Total	p value
Etiology (HCV/HBV)	70/30	63/16	20/7	39/3	189/56	
Sex (male/female)	55/44	45/32	15/12	22/20	137/108	
Age, years	51.4 ± 12.8	59.6 ± 14.0	59.6 ± 14.9	66.7 ± 11.6	57.7 ± 14.3	<0.001
Height, m	162.1 ± 8.2	165.3 ± 8.7	161.5 ± 7.5	160.1 ± 9.2	162.5 ± 8.4	NS
Weight, kg	60.7 ± 10.9	65.5 ± 14.7	59.4 ± 9.4	61.2 ± 14.2	61.7 ± 12.1	NS
Waist circumference, cm	82.8 ± 8.6	90.1 ± 14.1	87.9 ± 12.4	87.2 ± 10.6	85.7 ± 10.6	NS
Body mass index	23.1 ± 3.5	23.8 ± 4.2	22.8 ± 3.5	23.6 ± 3.7	23.3 ± 3.7	NS
AST, IU/l	43.6 ± 33.8	58.3 ± 48.2	63.3 ± 42.2	70.0 ± 47.2	54.0 ± 41.8	<0.001
ALT, IU/l	57.0 ± 63.3	69.6 ± 55.7	57.6 ± 46.7	59.7 ± 45.3	60.1 ± 56.6	NS
GGT, IU/l	42.3 ± 48.8	62.1 ± 70.1	45.2 ± 44.2	61.8 ± 86.6	50.4 ± 62.2	NS
ALP, IU/l	238.2 ± 83.4	266.6 ± 95.3	307.0 ± 169.8	376.7 ± 209.5	280.4 ± 141.4	<0.001
Total bilirubin, mg/dl	0.72 ± 0.49	0.92 ± 1.48	0.78 ± 0.58	1.09 ± 0.63	0.84 ± 0.82	<0.001
Total protein, g/dl	7.8 ± 7.1	7.2 ± 0.7	7.1 ± 0.9	7.1 ± 0.8	7.5 ± 4.9	NS
Serum albumin, g/dl	4.2 ± 0.4	4.1 ± 0.4	4.1 ± 0.7	3.6 ± 0.6	4.1 ± 0.5	<0.001
Gamma globulin, g/dl	1.4 ± 0.4	1.6 ± 0.4	1.7 ± 0.5	2.0 ± 0.5	1.6 ± 0.5	<0.001
Cholinesterase, IU/l	353.9 ± 99.8	288.3 ± 47.4	273.9 ± 76.5	157.4 ± 80.0	313.8 ± 105.0	<0.001
Total cholesterol, mg/dl	185.3 ± 32.7	172.2 ± 31.2	161.5 ± 34.9	149.7 ± 26.8	172.8 ± 34.4	<0.001
Prothrombin time, %	100.4 ± 11.7	95.8 ± 15.6	89.1 ± 14.9	76.6 ± 15.4	93.2 ± 16.4	<0.001
Platelets, $10^4/mm^3$	21.0 ± 6.0	15.7 ± 5.0	14.1 ± 4.7	10.6 ± 7.5	17.1 ± 7.3	<0.001
AST/ALT ratio	1.09 ± 0.92	1.01 ± 0.45	1.59 ± 1.46	1.33 ± 0.53	1.18 ± 0.88	0.001
APRI	5.49 ± 4.14	11.37 ± 13.68	12.52 ± 7.87	23.79 ± 26.23	11.05 ± 15.14	<0.001
FibroIndex	1.21 ± 0.45	1.78 ± 0.60	1.82 ± 0.55	2.31 ± 0.66	1.63 ± 0.70	<0.001
LFI	1.58 ± 0.67	2.03 ± 0.71	2.40 ± 0.64	2.86 ± 0.64	2.02 ± 0.82	<0.001
Total, n	99	77	27	42	245	

GGT = γ-Glutamyl transpeptidase; ALP = alkaline phosphatase.

showed a significant stepwise increase with severity of liver fibrosis ($p < 0.001$). However, there were a number of outliers in these serological markers (fig. 2).

Comparison between each F stage group was performed. Platelet count showed a significant decrease with severity of liver fibrosis between F0–F1 and F2, F0–F1 and F3, F0–F1 and F4, and F2 and F4. APRI showed a significant increase with severity of liver fibrosis between F0–F1 and F4, F2 and F4, and F3 and F4. FibroIndex showed a significant increase with severity of liver fibrosis between F0–F1 and F2, F0–F1 and F3, F0–F1 and F4, F2 and F4, and F3 and F4 (fig. 2).

Relationship between LFI and Pathological Liver Fibrosis

RTE was performed in all the enrolled patients. LFI was calculated as the median from 10 images. The median LFI in patients with F0–F1, F2, F3 and F4 stage fibrosis was 1.58, 2.03, 2.40 and 2.86, respectively, demonstrating a stepwise increase with increasing severity of liver fibrosis ($p < 0.001$). Comparison between each F stage group was performed. There was a significant increase between F0–F1 and F2, F0–F1 and F3, F0–F1 and F4, F2 and F4, and F3 and F4. The best cutoff of LFI for diagnosis of F2 or higher stage fibrosis (differentiating F2–F4 from F0–F1) was 2.05, and the accuracy was 73.0%. The best cutoff of LFI for diagnosis of F3 or higher stage fibrosis (differentiating F3–F4 from F0–F2) was 2.28, and the accuracy was 79.6%. The best cutoff of LFI for diagnosis of F4 stage fibrosis (differentiating F4 from F0–F3) was 2.36, and the accuracy was 78.3 (table 2).

Correlation with LFI and Serum Markers

The AUROC of the LFI, platelet count, AST/ALT ratio, APRI and FibroIndex for predicting F2 or higher stage fibrosis (F0–F1 vs. F2–F4) was 0.800, 0.832, 0.646, 0.820 and 0.853, respectively. Similarly, the AUROC for predicting F3 or higher stage fibrosis (F0–F2 vs. F3–F4) was 0.865, 0.824, 0.708, 0.789 and 0.828, respectively.

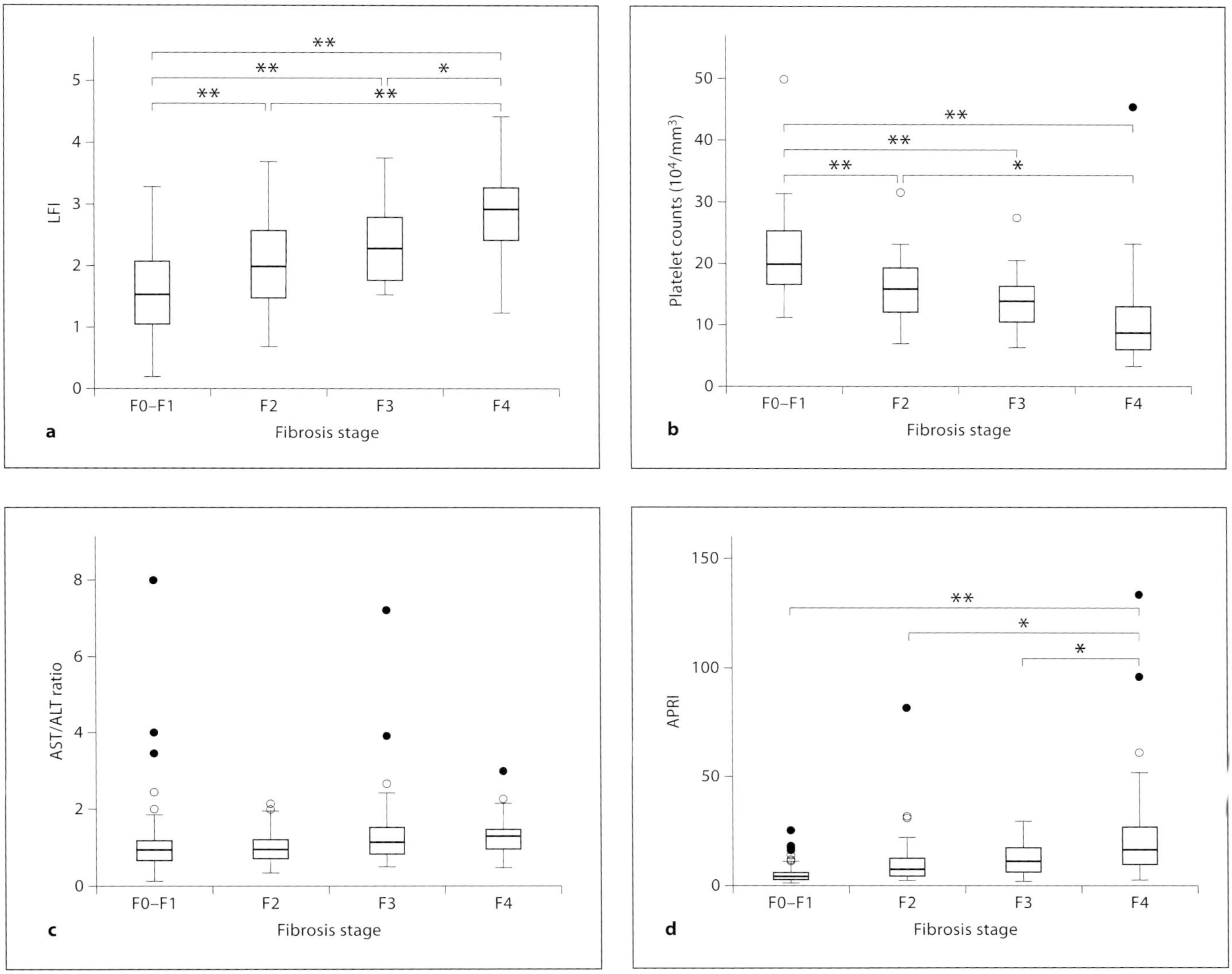

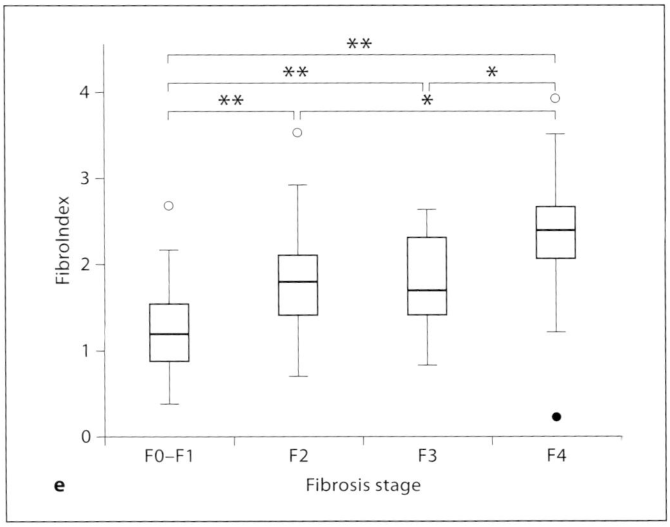

Fig. 2. LFI and serological markers for each fibrosis stage. **a** LFI for each fibrosis stage. The lines through the middle of the boxes represent the medians. The top and bottom of each box represents the 1st and 3rd quartiles. The length of the box represents the interquartile range within which 50% of the values were located. F2 versus F3 did not differ significantly ($p = 0.066$), whereas there were significant differences in all the other combinations of stages. There was no outlier. **b** Platelet counts for each fibrosis stage. Many outliers (open circles) were present. Black circles are extreme outliers, representing a case with a value of more than three times the height of the box. **c** AST/ALT ratio for each fibrosis stage. There were no significant differences with each fibrosis stage and many extreme outliers were present. **d** APRI for each fibrosis stage; many extreme outliers were present. **e** FibroIndex for each fibrosis stage; many outliers were present. * $p < 0.05$, ** $p < 0.001$, comparing between each fibrosis stage.

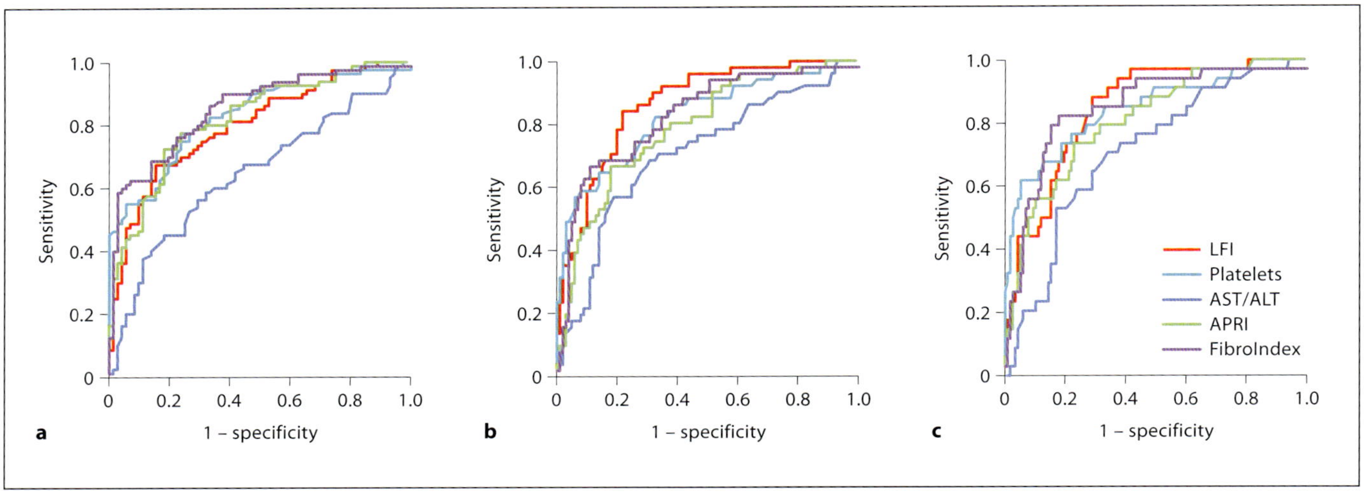

Fig. 3. a ROC curve of the LFI, platelet count, AST/ALT ratio, APRI, and FibroIndex for predicting F2 stage or higher fibrosis (F0–F1 vs. F2–F4). **b** ROC of predicting F3 stage or higher fibrosis. **c** ROC of predicting stage F4 fibrosis.

Table 2. Sensitivity, specificity, positive predictive value, negative predictive value and accuracy of cutoff values of LFI for predicting hepatic fibrosis stage

	Fibrosis stage		
	F0–F1 vs. F2–F4	F0–F2 vs. F3–F4	F0–F3 vs. F4
AUROC	0.800	0.865	0.846
Cutoff value	2.049	2.278	2.357
Sensitivity, %	70.0	78.4	73.5
Specificity, %	76.4	80.2	79.7
Positive predictive value, %	76.7	66.7	51.0
Negative predictive value, %	69.6	88.0	91.3
Accuracy, %	73.0	79.6	78.3

Table 3. AUROC of LFI and several serological makers for predicting liver fibrosis stage

	LFI	Platelets	AST/ALT	APRI	FibroIndex
F0–F1 vs. F2–F4	0.800	0.832	0.646	0.820	0.853
F0–F2 vs. F3–F4	0.865	0.824	0.708	0.789	0.828
F0–F3 vs. F4	0.846	0.840	0.710	0.809	0.850

For diagnosis of cirrhosis (F0–F3 vs. F4), AUROC was 0.846, 0.840, 0.710, 0.809 and 0.850, respectively (table 3, fig. 3). Regardless of the degree of fibrosis progression, RTE has a very good diagnostic capability for liver fibrosis.

Discussion

There is a variety of methods for performing elastography. FibroScan, virtual-touch tissue quantification and shear wave elastography measure the velocity of propagation of the shear wave, which is displayed as elastic modulus or velocity. As the liver becomes hard, the speed of propagation increases. However, the hardness of the liver is also affected by inflammation, jaundice and congestion, as well as fibrosis. FibroScan has been most frequently used in clinical practice to evaluate advanced fibrosis without liver biopsy. However, FibroScan cannot be performed in patients with ascites, narrow intercostal space or severe obesity. Furthermore, it has the disadvantage of low accuracy because there is no B-mode.

RTE displays in real time the relative strain of the tissue by measuring its displacement and does not have the limitations of FibroScan. In the mammary gland, thyroid and prostate, the relative degree of elastic modulus can distinguish malignant space-occupying lesions [13, 14, 20]. As mentioned previously, as liver fibrosis progresses, the blue portion of the strain image tends to increase in RTE [21]. Shiina et al. [22] have indicated that this pattern of strain images is related to the fibrous structure changes of fibrosis. Several previous studies have focused on the diagnostic accuracy of RTE for liver fibrosis. There are few reports representing a poor accuracy of liver fibrosis. However, the reason for the poor diagnostic accuracy may be the lack of experience of the examiners. To the best of our knowledge, we have been one of the first groups worldwide to perform RTE in patients with liver fibrosis [18, 21, 23, 24]. It is slightly difficult to visualize strain images well. Artifacts such as multiple reflections at the surface of the liver, echo-free areas by thick blood vessels, ribs and lungs, and lack of penetration should be avoided if possible. These are important issues when performing RTE. Although manipulative pressure is used during RTE of the mammary gland and thyroid gland, we performed RTE of the liver without using such pressure. If manipulative pressure is too strong, there is a possibility that the elastic relationship will vary due to the elastic nonlinearity. In addition, there is a possibility that the pressure is not uniformly transmitted to the liver. On the other hand, the liver is deformed slightly by the steady rhythm of the heartbeat. Good images can be obtained merely by light application of the probe to the right intercostal region. Furthermore, because manipulative pressure is not used, human error can be minimized.

LFI in stage F2 fibrosis did not significantly differ from that in stage F3, whereas in all other combinations of stages there were significant differences. The AUROC for prediction of ≥F4 and ≥F2 of LFI was higher than that of serological markers. Our study confirmed that RTE is useful for distinguishing not only advanced fibrosis patients but also mild fibrosis patients from others. Moreover, our study showed that RTE can be performed in all cases, with good discrimination of each fibrosis stage.

In summary, we demonstrated a convenient and noninvasive tool, RTE, for relative strain imaging of the liver. We found that LFI measured by RTE is a useful predictive factor for diagnosis of liver fibrosis stage in patients with chronic viral hepatitis. Our study was based on the gold standard of diagnosis by liver biopsy; therefore, there was a possibility of sampling error. Further studies are desirable on a large number of patients with diagnosis of fibrosis using surgical specimens.

Disclosure Statement

The authors declare that no conflicts of interests exist.

References

1 Nord HJ: Biopsy diagnosis of cirrhosis: blind percutaneous versus guided direct vision techniques – a review. Gastrointest Endosc 1982;28:102–104.

2 Regev A, Berho M, Jeffers LJ, Milikowski C, Molina EG, Pyrsopoulos NT, Feng ZZ, Reddy KR, Schiff ER: Sampling error and intraobserver variation in liver biopsy in patients with chronic HCV infection. Am J Gastroenterol 2002;97:2614–2618.

3 Bedossa P, Dargere D, Paradis V: Sampling variability of liver fibrosis in chronic hepatitis C. Hepatology 2003;38:1449–1457.

4 Joo I, Choi BI: New paradigm for management of hepatocellular carcinoma by imaging. Liver Cancer 2012;1:94–109.

5 Kim DY, Kim SU, Park JY, Ahn SH, Song KJ, Han KH: FibroScan based risk estimation of HBV-related HCC occurrence: development and validation of a predictive model. Liver Cancer 2012;1:123.

6 Sandrin L, Fourquet B, Hasquenoph JM, Yon S, Fournier C, Mal F, Christidis C, Ziol M, Poulet B, Kazemi F, Beaugrand M, Palau R: Transient elastography: a new noninvasive method for assessment of hepatic fibrosis. Ultras Med Biol 2003;29:1705–1713.

7 Friedrich-Rust M, Wunder K, Kriener S, Sotoudeh F, Richter S, Bojunga J, Herrmann E, Poynard T, Dietrich CF, Vermehren J, Zeuzem S, Sarrazin C: Liver fibrosis in viral hepatitis: noninvasive assessment with acoustic radiation force impulse imaging versus transient elastography. Radiology 2009;252:595–604.

8 Ferraioli G, Tinelli C, Dal Bello B, Zicchetti M, Filice G, Filice C: Accuracy of real-time shear wave elastography for assessing liver fibrosis in chronic hepatitis C: a pilot study. Hepatology 2012, E-pub ahead of print.

9 Arena U, Vizzutti F, Corti G, Ambu S, Stasi C, Bresci S, Moscarella S, Boddi V, Petrarca A, Laffi G, Marra F, Pinzani M: Acute viral hepatitis increases liver stiffness values measured by transient elastography. Hepatology 2008;47:380–384.

10 Cobbold JF, Taylor-Robinson SD: Transient elastography in acute hepatitis: all that's stiff is not fibrosis. Hepatology 2008;47:370–372.

11 Millonig G, Reimann FM, Friedrich S, Fonouni H, Mehrabi A, Buchler MW, Seitz HK, Mueller S: Extrahepatic cholestasis increases liver stiffness (FibroScan) irrespective of fibrosis. Hepatology 2008;48:1718–1723.

12 Colli A, Pozzoni P, Berzuini A, Gerosa A, Canovi C, Molteni EE, Barbarini M, Bonino F, Prati D: Decompensated chronic heart failure: increased liver stiffness measured by means of transient elastography. Radiology 2010;257:872–878.

13 Itoh A, Ueno E, Tohno E, Kamma H, Takahashi H, Shiina T, Yamakawa M, Matsumura T: Breast disease: clinical application of US elastography for diagnosis. Radiology 2006;239:341–350.

14 Fukunari N: More accurate and sensitive diagnosis for thyroid tumors with elastography – detection and differential diagnosis of thyroid cancers. MEDIX Suppl. 2007. http://www.hitachi-medical.co.jp/tech/medix/pdf/supple/sup_05.pdf.

15 Williams AL, Hoofnagle JH: Ratio of serum aspartate to alanine aminotransferase in chronic hepatitis: relationship to cirrhosis. Gastroenterology 1988;95:734–739.

16 Wai CT, Greenson JK, Fontana RJ, Kalbfleisch JD, Marrero JA, Conjeevaram HS, Lok AS: A simple noninvasive index can predict both significant fibrosis and cirrhosis in patients with chronic hepatitis C. Hepatology 2003;38:518–526.

17 Koda M, Matunaga Y, Kawakami M, Kishimoto Y, Suou T, Murawaki Y: FibroIndex, a practical index for predicting significant fibrosis in patients with chronic hepatitis C. Hepatology 2007;45:297–306.

18 Tatsumi C, Kudo M, Ueshima K, Kitai S, Ishikawa E, Yada N, Hagiwara S, Inoue T, Minami Y, Chung H, Maekawa K, Fujimoto K, Kato M, Tonomura A, Mitake T, Shiina T: Non-invasive evaluation of hepatic fibrosis for type C chronic hepatitis. Intervirology 2010;53:76–81.

19 Fujimoto K, Kato M, Tonomura A, Yada N, Tatsumi C, Oshita M, Wada S, Ueshima K, Ishida T, Furuta T, Yamasaki M, Tsujimoto M, Motoki M, Mitake T, Shiina T, Kudo M, Hayashi N: Non-invasive evaluation method of the liver fibrosis using real-time tissue elastograpy: usefulness of judgment liver fibrosis stage by liver fibrosis index (LF index). Kanzo 2010;59:539–541.

20 Miyanaga N, Akaza H, Yamakawa M, Oikawa T, Sekido N, Hinotsu S, Kawai K, Shimazui T, Shiina T: Tissue elasticity imaging for diagnosis of prostate cancer: a preliminary report. Int J Urol 2006;13:1514–1518.

21 Fujimoto K, Wada S, Oshita M, Kato M, Tonomura A, Mitake T: Non-invasive evaluation of hepatic fibrosis in patients with chronic hepatitis C using elastography. MEDIX Suppl. 2007. http://www.hitachi-medical.co.jp/tech/medix/pdf/supple/sup_07.pdf.

22 Shiina T, Maki T, Yamakawa M, Mitake T, Kudo M, Fujimoto K: Mechanical model analysis for quantitative evaluation of liver fibrosis based on ultrasound tissue elasticity imaging. Jpn J Appl Phys 2012; DOI: 10.1143/JJAP.51.07GF11.

23 Morikawa H, Fukuda K, Kobayashi S, Fujii H, Iwai S, Enomoto M, Tamori A, Sakaguchi H, Kawada N: Real-time tissue elastography as a tool for the noninvasive assessment of liver stiffness in patients with chronic hepatitis C. J Gastroenterol 2011; 46:350–358.

24 Tatsumi C, Kudo M, Ueshima K, Kitai S, Takahashi S, Inoue T, Minami Y, Chung H, Maekawa K, Fujimoto K, Akiko T, Takeshi M: Noninvasive evaluation of hepatic fibrosis using serum fibrotic markers, transient elastography (FibroScan) and real-time tissue elastography. Intervirology 2008;51 (suppl 1):27–33.

Oncology

Oncology 2013;84(suppl 1):21–27
DOI: 10.1159/000345885

Published online: February 20, 2013

Role of Gadolinium-Ethoxybenzyl-Diethylenetriamine Pentaacetic Acid-Enhanced Magnetic Resonance Imaging in the Management of Hepatocellular Carcinoma: Consensus at the Symposium of the 48th Annual Meeting of the Liver Cancer Study Group of Japan

Masatoshi Kudo[a] Osamu Matsui[b] Michiie Sakamoto[c] Azusa Kitao[b] Tonsok Kim[e] Shun-ichi Ariizumi[d] Tomoaki Ichikawa[f] Satoshi Kobayashi[b] Yasuharu Imai[g] Namiki Izumi[h] Yasunari Fujinaga[i] Shigeki Arii[j]

[a]Department of Gastroenterology and Hepatology, Kinki University School of Medicine, Osakasayama, [b]Department of Radiology, Kanazawa University Graduate School of Medical Science, Kanazawa, [c]Department of Pathology, Keio University School of Medicine, and [d]Department of Surgery, Institute of Gastroenterology, Tokyo Women's Medical University, Tokyo, [e]Department of Radiology, Osaka University Graduate School of Medicine, Osaka, [f]Department of Radiology, University of Yamanashi, Yamanashi, [g]Department of Gastroenterology, Ikeda Municipal Hospital, Ikeda, [h]Division of Gastroenterology and Hepatology, Musashino Red Cross Hospital, Musashino, [i]Department of Radiology, Shinshu University School of Medicine, Matsumoto, and [j]Department of Surgery, Hamamatsu Rosai Hospital, Hamamatsu, Japan

Key Words

Hepatocellular carcinoma · EOB-MRI · Expert consensus

Abstract

We summarize here the consensus reached at the Symposium of the 48th Annual Meeting of the Liver Cancer Study Group of Japan held in Kanazawa on July 20th and 21st, 2012, on the role of gadolinium-ethoxybenzyl-diethylenetriamine pentaacetic acid-enhanced magnetic resonance imaging (EOB-MRI) in the management of hepatocellular carcinoma (HCC). Currently, dynamic CT is the first choice of imaging modality when HCC is suspected. EOB-MRI is useful for differentiation and definitive diagnosis of HCC when dynamic CT/MRI does not show conclusive findings for HCC. In addition, contrast- enhanced ultrasound with Sonazoid is useful for making a decision on whether or not to treat a hypovascular lesion <1 cm when the nodules are shown with low intensity in the hepatocyte phase of EOB-MRI. Furthermore, EOB-MRI should be performed in selected cases of HCC ultrahigh-risk groups every 3–4 months, or EOB-MRI should be performed at least once at the first visit in all HCC ultrahigh-risk groups.

Introduction

Gadolinium-ethoxybenzyl-diethylenetriamine pentaacetic acid (Gd-EOB-DTPA; Primovist, Bayer Healthcare, Leverkusen, Germany) [1–5] has been available in Japan as a magnetic resonance imaging (MRI) contrast agent for more than 4 years since its release in January 2008. This contrast agent, consisting of Gd-DTPA conjugated with an ethoxybenzyl (EOB) group, has the characteristics of both an extracellular Gd contrast agent and a hepatocyte-specific contrast agent. Because Gd-EOB-DTPA-enhanced MRI (EOB-MRI) allow for the observa-

KARGER

Fax +41 61 306 12 34
E-Mail karger@karger.com
www.karger.com

0030–2414/13/0847–0021$38.00/0

Accessible online at:
www.karger.com/ocl

Masatoshi Kudo, MD, PhD
Division of Gastroenterology and Hepatology, Department of Internal Medicine
Kinki University School of Medicine
377-2 Ohno-Higashi, Osakasayama, Osaka 589-8511 (Japan)
E-Mail m-kudo@med.kindai.ac.jp

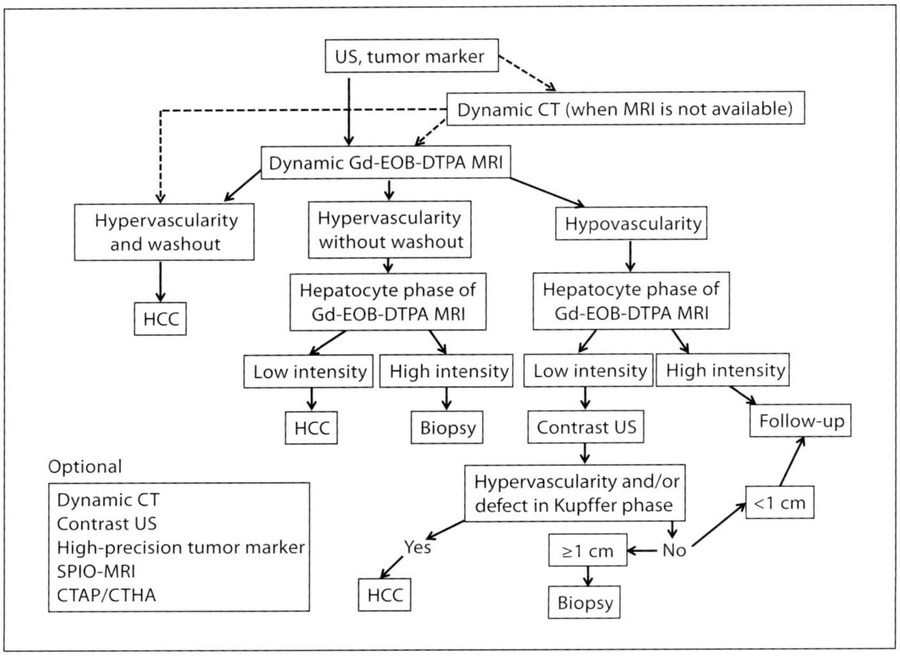

Color version available online

Fig. 1. New diagnostic algorithm proposed by the research group (headed by Shigeki Arii) supported by the Japan Ministry of Health, Labour and Welfare.

tion of blood flow in hepatocellular carcinoma (HCC) and the function of hepatocyte, diagnosis made by EOB-MRI is reportedly superior to diagnosis of hepatic blood flow either by dynamic computed tomography (CT) using multi-detector CT, dynamic MRI using an extracellular Gd contrast agent, or functional diagnosis of hepatic Kupffer cells by superparamagnetic iron oxide (SPIO)-MRI [6–13]. EOB-MRI is highly capable of detecting not only typical hypervascular HCC but also early-stage hypovascular HCC [11–13], greatly influencing early diagnosis and treatment for HCC. However, MRI is not as widespread as CT and it takes longer to complete EOB-MRI than dynamic CT, thus limiting the number of EOB-MRI scans performed in daily clinical practice.

Based on this background, the Symposium of the 48th Annual Meeting of the Liver Cancer Study Group of Japan was held on July 20th, 2012, to address the role of EOB-MRI in the management of HCC. Here, we report the consensus reached using a key-pad answering system in the meeting. Votes were cast by 144 experts specialized in internal medicine (57%), radiology (24%), surgery (12%), pathology (4%) and other fields (3%). This report describes consensus of current clinical practice for patients with HCC in Japan. The consensuses that achieved more than 67% agreement were summarized as 'consensus statements'. Furthermore, issues obtaining more than 50% agreement were summarized as 'informative statements'.

Novel Diagnostic Algorithm Proposed for the Management of HCC

In Japan, HCC diagnostic algorithms have been proposed in the EBM-based 'HCC Clinical Practice Guidelines' [14] and the 'HCC Clinical Practice Manual' [15] based on EBM plus consensus reached by HCC experts. The algorithm in the 'HCC Clinical Practice Manual' reflects Japan's sophisticated approach to the detection of early HCC and is in line with the actual clinical situation; however, the algorithm is somewhat complicated to use as a clinical practice guideline. Moreover, there is an increasing need to develop a simple HCC diagnostic algorithm centered on EOB-MRI, owing to its good diagnostic capability, simplicity and highly objective nature. Accordingly, a new HCC diagnostic algorithm was proposed in March 2012 by the research group (headed by Dr. Shigeki Arii) funded by the Ministry of Health, Labour and Welfare for the 'development of molecular markers and diagnostic imaging systems for the early detection of HCC' (fig. 1).

This algorithm basically recommends the implementation of EOB-MRI in cases where HCC is suspected by B-mode ultrasound findings and tumor marker measurements. The diagnosis of HCC is made when a nodular lesion is hypervascular in the arterial phase and washed out in the late phase on EOB-MRI images. HCC is also diagnosed when nodular lesions are hypervascular

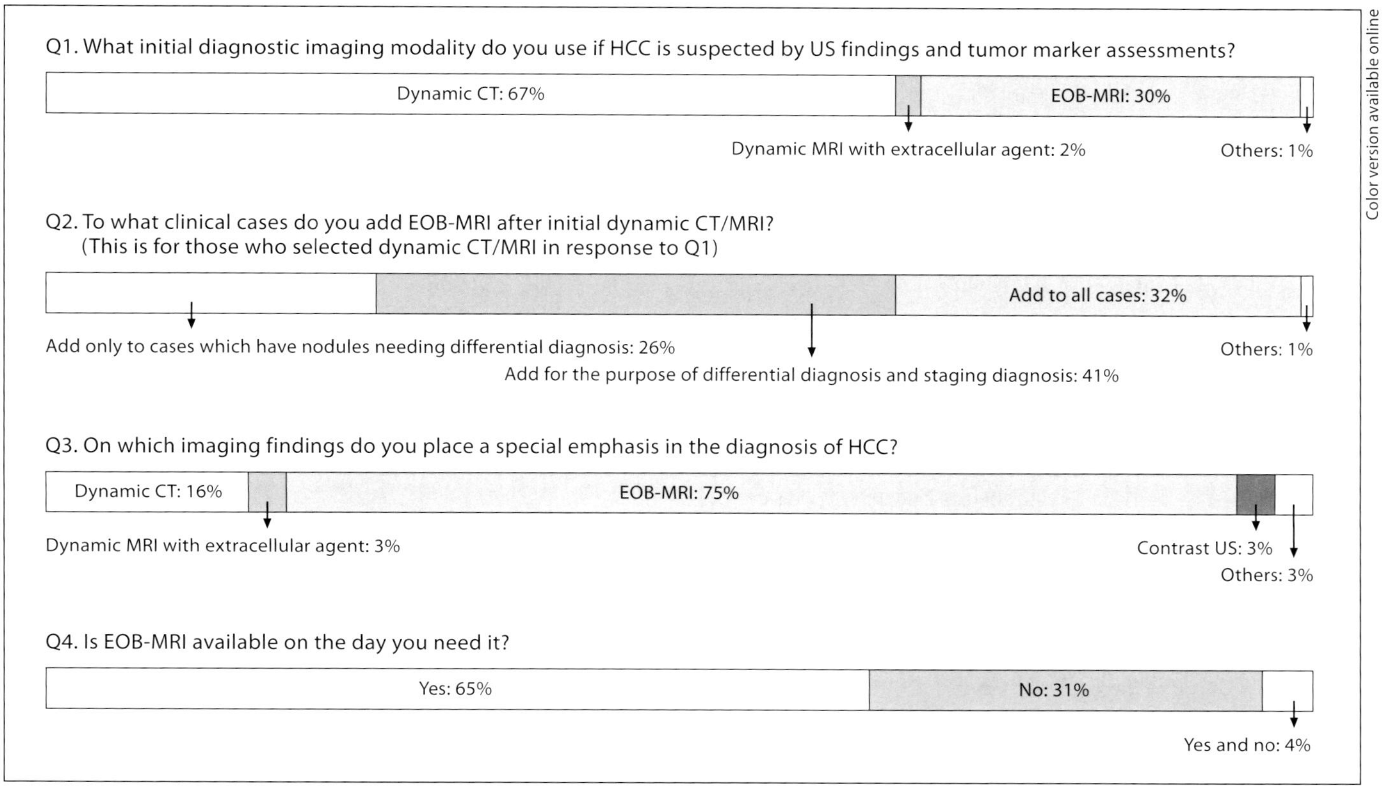

Fig. 2. Questions 1–4 and responses.

in the arterial phase and hypointense in the hepatocyte phase of EOB-MRI, even if it is difficult to determine the degree of washout in the portal phase (with the exclusion of hemangioma by another imaging modality). When hypervascular nodular lesions are hyperintense in the hepatocyte phase on EOB-MRI imaging, they are difficult to diagnose as HCC, but can be diagnosed as HCC when the capsule or mosaic structure is apparent. Biopsy is recommended if the diagnosis is not definitive.

On the other hand, if nodular lesions are hypovascular in the arterial phase and hypointense in the hepatocyte phase on EOB-MRI images, contrast-enhanced ultrasonography (US) using Sonazoid is required to confirm hypervascularity or defects in the Kupffer phase in order to make a definitive diagnosis of HCC. If hypervascularity or defects in the Kupffer phase are absent, lesions ≥1 cm in diameter should be biopsied and those <1 cm need to be followed up. Follow-up observations are also recommended for nodular lesions that are hypovascular in the arterial phase and hyperintense in the hepatocyte phase on EOB-MRI images. Furthermore, institutions unable to conduct MRI as initial diagnostic imaging need to perform dynamic CT first, followed by EOB-MRI as the recommended diagnostic method. CT arterial portography/CT hepatic arteriography (CTAP/CTHA), SPIO-MRI and high-precision tumor marker assessments should be performed as needed at each institution. At the symposium, we evaluated HCC management on the basis of this algorithm and voted for the consensus.

Consensus Voting Results

Selection of Diagnostic Imaging Modality: Questions 1–4

When HCC is suspected based on US and tumor marker findings, 67% of physicians would select dynamic CT as the initial diagnostic imaging, 30% EOB-MRI and 2% dynamic MRI. When those who had selected dynamic CT/MRI were asked to which clinical cases they would add EOB-MRI, 41% selected 'cases requiring differential diagnosis and staging' and 32% responded with 'all cases'. When asked on what imaging findings they would place a special emphasis in the diagnosis of HCC, 75% of physi-

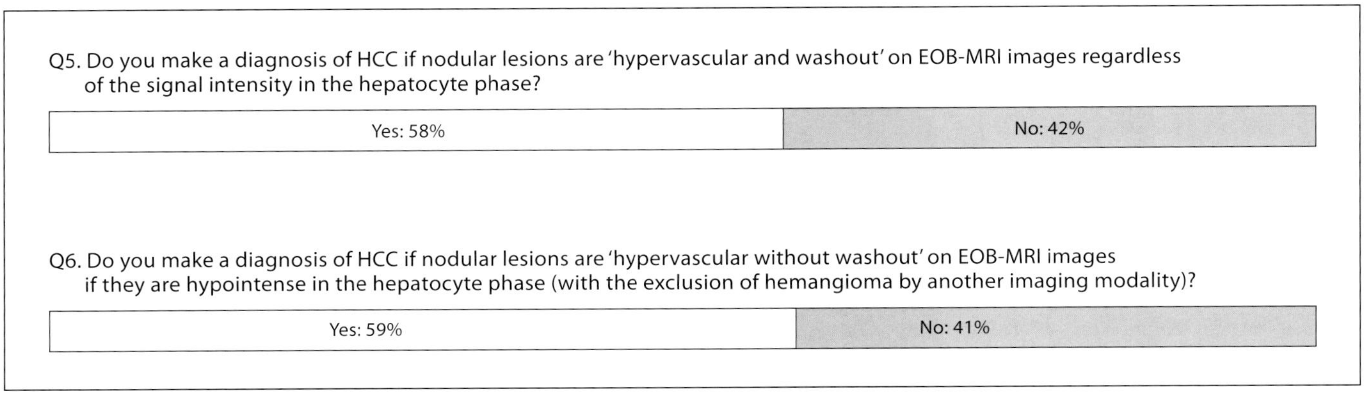

Color version available online

Fig. 3. Questions 5–6 and responses.

cians selected EOB-MRI and 16% dynamic CT. However, because only 65% of physicians answered that EOB-MRI was available on the day they needed it, availability of MRI at each institution might have affected the selection of initial diagnostic imaging modality (fig. 2).

Diagnosis of Hypervascular HCC by EOB-MRI: Questions 5–6

'HCC is diagnosed if nodular lesions are hypervascular in the arterial phase and washed out in the portal/equilibrium phase on EOB-MRI images regardless of the signal intensity in the hepatocyte phase' was selected by 58% of physicians. Similarly, 'HCC is diagnosed if nodular lesions are hypervascular in the arterial phase and hypointense in the hepatocyte phase of EOB-MRI even if no washout is observed (with the exclusion of hemangioma by another imaging modality)' was selected by 59% of physicians. We think that the answer to this question was affected by the fact that the patients in question are not restricted to those with cirrhosis, that washout is interpreted differently between EOB-MRI and dynamic MRI using extracellular Gd contrast agents, and that some pseudotumors such as arterioportal shunt exhibit low signals in the hepatocyte phase (fig. 3).

Diagnosis and Treatment of Hypovascular HCC: Questions 7–14

When asked if they would treat hypovascular nodular lesions ≥1.5 cm in diameter with hypointense signals in the hepatocyte phase of EOB-MRI, 55% of physicians voted for 'treat based on the results of additional imaging', 23% selected 'treat if biopsy confirms cancer', 17% chose 'treat with no additional imaging' and only 5% selected 'assign to follow-up observation'. As additional imaging, 52% of physicians would select contrast-enhanced US with Sonazoid and 45% CTAP/CTHA. When nodular lesions are ≥1.0 cm but <1.5 cm, 72% would 'treat based on the results of additional imaging', 18% would 'treat if biopsy confirms cancer', 5% would 'treat with no additional imaging' and another 5% would 'assign to follow-up observation'. For nodular lesions <1.0 cm, 9% of physicians would consider the option 'assign to follow-up observations'. In summary, a certain number of physicians would treat hypointense nodular lesions in the hepatocyte phase even if the lesions were hypovascular.

When asked about the most appropriate diagnostic imaging to perform when deciding whether to follow up hypovascular nodular lesions with hypointense signals in the hepatocyte phase of EOB-MRI, 63% of physicians selected EOB-MRI, 9% chose contrast-enhanced US with Sonazoid, 6% nominated dynamic CT, 2% indicated dynamic MRI and 20% suggested combinations of these imaging modalities. Physicians considered 6 months (56%) and 3 months (41%) to be the most appropriate interval for follow-up observations (fig. 4).

HCC Screening: Questions 15–17

When asked whether EOB-MRI should be performed for ultrahigh-risk groups (patients with cirrhosis due to hepatitis B or C) as a screening tool, 49% of physicians selected 'in all cases' and 42% 'depending on the case'. To clarify the definition of 'a screening tool', physicians were further asked whether such high-risk individuals should undergo EOB-MRI every 3–4 months: overwhelmingly, 71% selected 'depending on the case'. In addition, the majority of physicians (83%) answered 'in all cases' to the question of whether 'EOB-MRI should be used at least once in patients at ultrahigh-risk for HCC' (fig. 5).

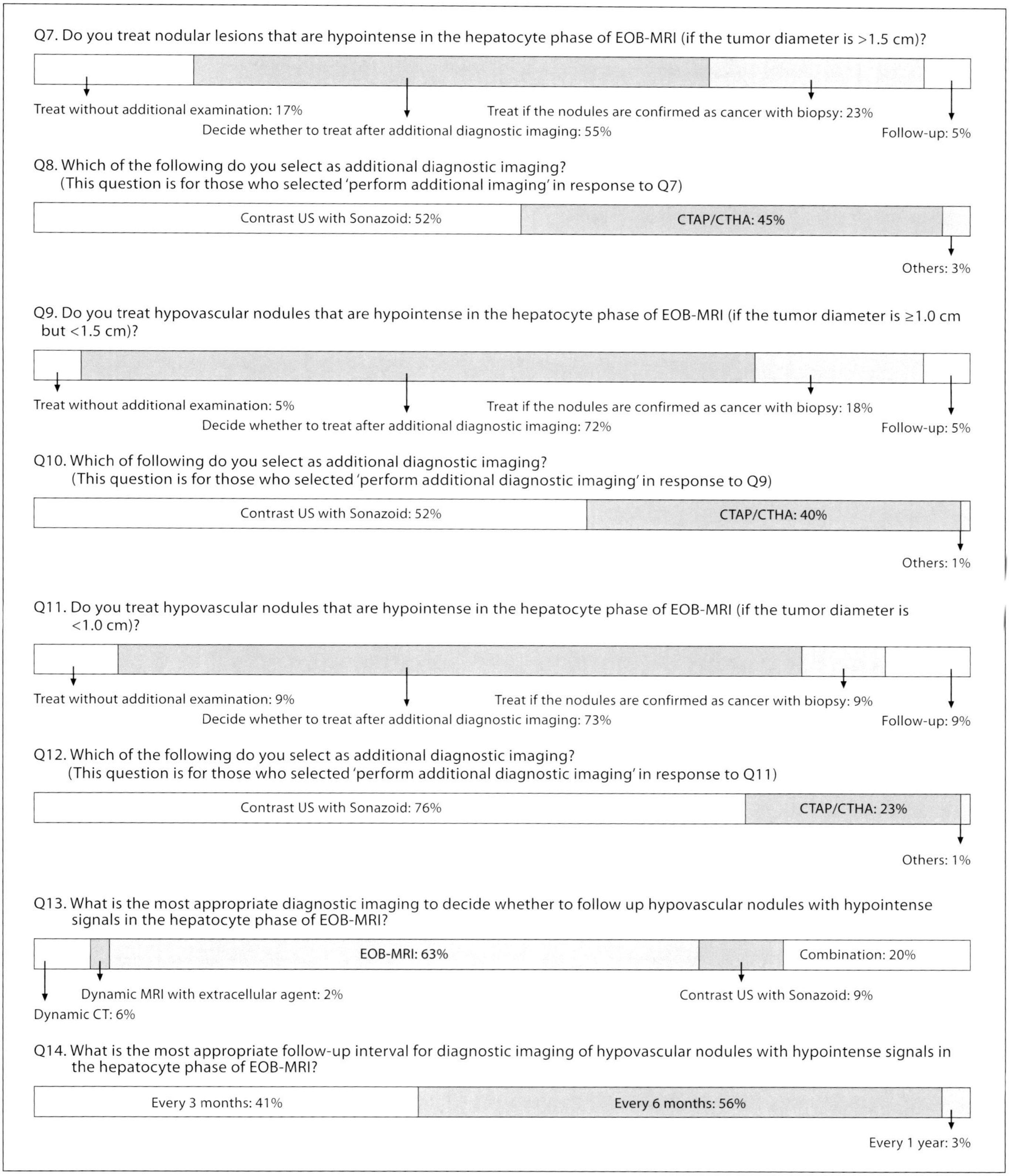

Color version available online

Fig. 4. Questions 7–14 and responses.

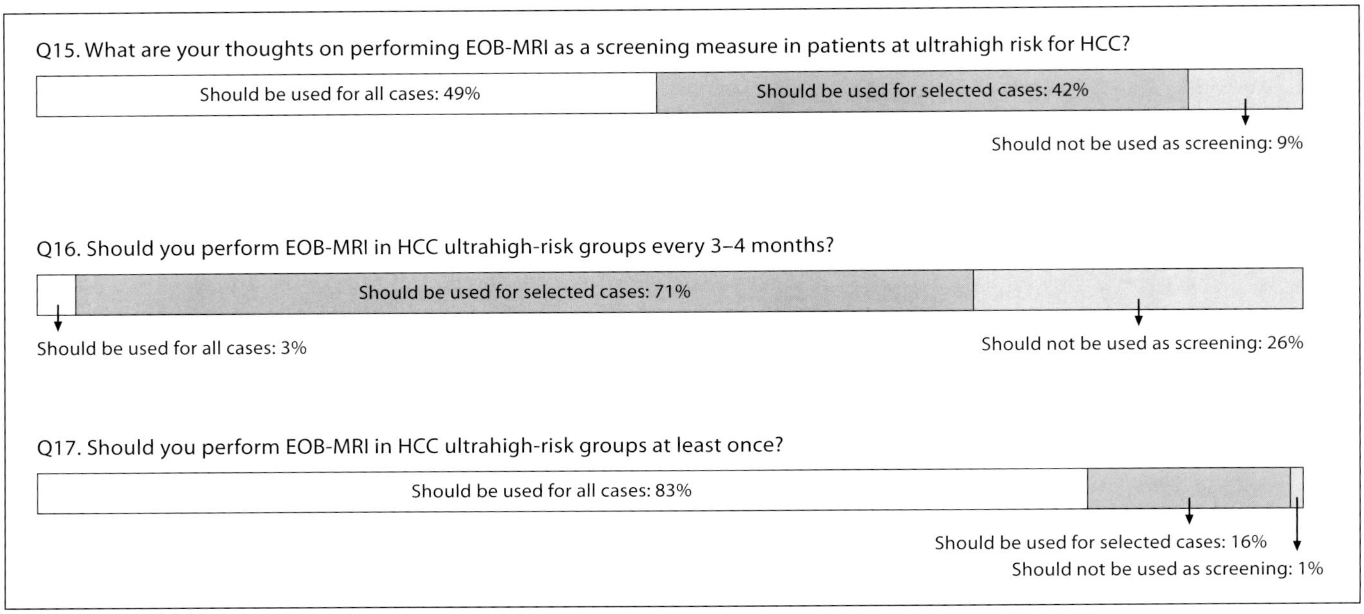

Color version available online

Fig. 5. Questions 15–17 and responses.

Consensus Statements

(1) Currently, dynamic CT is the first choice of imaging modality when HCC is suspected (agreement: 67%).
(2) EOB-MRI is useful for differentiation and definitive diagnosis of HCC when dynamic CT/MRI does not show conclusive findings for HCC (agreement: 75%).
(3) Contrast-enhanced US with Sonazoid is useful for making a decision on whether or not to treat hypovascular lesions <1 cm when the nodules are shown with low intensity in the hepatocyte phase (agreement: 76%).
(4) EOB-MRI should be performed in selected cases of HCC ultrahigh-risk groups every 3–4 months (agreement: 71%).
(5) EOB-MRI should be performed at least once in all HCC ultrahigh-risk groups (agreement: 83%).

Informative Statements

(1) HCC can be confirmed by EOB-MRI when nodular lesions show arterial hypervascularity with venous washout (agreement: 58%).
(2) HCC can be confirmed by EOB-MRI when nodular lesions show arterial hypervascularity with low intensity on hepatocyte phase (agreement: 59%).
(3) Contrast-enhanced US with Sonazoid is useful for making a decision on whether or not to treat nodules >1 cm when the hypovascular nodules are shown with low intensity in the hepatocyte phase of EOB-MRI (agreement: 59%).
(4) EOB-MRI is the most appropriate diagnostic tool to decide whether to treat or to follow up hypovascular nodules with hypointense in the hepatocyte phase EOB-MRI (agreement: 63%).
(5) Hypovascular nodules with hypointense signals in the hepatocyte phase of EOB-MRI should be followed up every 6 months (agreement: 56%).

Conclusion

The above results clearly show that EOB-MRI has become a crucial diagnostic imaging tool for HCC despite the problems associated with insufficient MRI availability. It is also clear that it is considered that hypointense nodular lesions in the hepatocyte phase on EOB-MRI images should be treated, even if the nodule is hypovascular, in current clinical practice in Japan.

Disclosure Statement

This symposium was sponsored by Bayer Yakuhin Ltd., Osaka, Japan.

References

1 Ricke J, Seidensticker M, Mohnike K: Noninvasive diagnosis of hepatocellular carcinoma in cirrhotic liver: current guidelines and future prospects for radiological imaging. Liver Cancer 2012;1:51–58.

2 Choi D: Imaging diagnosis of very small hepatocellular carcinoma in Gd-EOB-DTPA-enhanced and diffusion-weighted MRI. Liver Cancer 2012;1:115.

3 Lee JM, Phongkitrarun S, Bergmann K, Jeong M, Liamsuwa S, Luong B: Effectiveness of using Gd-EOB-DTPA-enhanced MRI for confirmation of hepatocellular carcinoma in Thailand and Korea as compared to extracellular contrast media-enhanced MRI and 3-phase MD-CT. Liver Cancer 2012;1:126.

4 Min YW, Paik SW, Gwak GY, Paik YH, Choi MS, Lee JH, et al: Utility of gadoxetic acid-enhanced MRI in the surveillance for postoperative recurrence of hepatocellular carcinoma. Liver Cancer 2012;1:129.

5 Choi JI, Jang HY, Lee YJ: Diagnostic accurary of gadoxetic acid enhanced magnetic resonance imaging in predicting the appropriateness of a transplant recipient based on the Milan criteria. Liver Cancer, in press.

6 Di Martino M, Marin D, Guerrisi A, Baski M, Galati F, Rossi M, et al: Intraindividual comparison of gadoxetate disodium-enhanced MR imaging and 64-section multidetector CT in the detection of hepatocellular carcinoma in patients with cirrhosis. Radiology 2010;256:806–816.

7 Haradome H, Grazioli L, Tinti R, Morone M, Motosugi U, Sano K, et al: Additional value of gadoxetic acid-DTPA-enhanced hepatobiliary phase MR imaging in the diagnosis of early-stage hepatocellular carcinoma: comparison with dynamic triple-phase multidetector CT imaging. J Magn Reson Imaging 2011;34:69–78.

8 Onishi H, Kim T, Imai Y, Hori M, Nagano H, Nakaya Y, et al: Hypervascular hepatocellular carcinomas: detection with gadoxetate disodium-enhanced MR imaging and multiphasic multidetector CT. Eur Radiol 2012;22:845–854.

9 Park G, Kim YK, Kim CS, Yu HC, Hwang SB: Diagnostic efficacy of gadoxetic acid-enhanced MRI in the detection of hepatocellular carcinomas: comparison with gadopentetate dimeglumine. Br J Radiol 2010;83:1010–1016.

10 Kim YK, Kim CS, Han YM, Park G, Hwang SB, Yu HC: Comparison of gadoxetic acid-enhanced MRI and superparamagnetic iron oxide-enhanced MRI for the detection of hepatocellular carcinoma. Clin Radiol 2010;65:358–365.

11 Okada M, Imai Y, Kim T, Kogita S, Takamura M, Kumano S, et al: Comparison of enhancement patterns of histologically confirmed hepatocellular carcinoma between gadoxetate- and ferucarbotran-enhanced magnetic resonance imaging. J Magn Reson Imaging 2010;32:903–913.

12 Kogita S, Imai Y, Okada M, Kim T, Onishi H, Takamura M, et al: Gd-EOB-DTPA-enhanced magnetic resonance images of hepatocellular carcinoma: correlation with histological grading and portal blood flow. Eur Radiol 2010;20:2405–2413.

13 Sano K, Ichikawa T, Motosugi U, Sou H, Muhi AM, Matsuda M, et al: Imaging study of early hepatocellular carcinoma: usefulness of gadoxetic acid-enhanced MR imaging. Radiology 2011;261:834–844.

14 Makuuchi M, Kokudo N, Arii S, Igaki H, Ikai I, Kaneko S, et al: Surveillance algorithm and diagnostic algorithm for hepatocellular carcinoma. Hepatology Research 2010;40(suppl 1):1–144.

15 Kudo M, Izumi N, Kokudo N, Matsui O, Sakamoto M, Nakashima O, et al: Management of hepatocellular carcinoma in Japan: Consensus-Based Clinical Practice Guidelines proposed by the Japan Society of Hepatology (JSH) 2010 updated version. Dig Dis 2011;29:339–364.

Oncology

Oncology 2013;84(suppl 1):28–33
DOI: 10.1159/000345886

Published online: February 20, 2013

Transcatheter Arterial Chemoembolization for Unresectable Hepatocellular Carcinoma: Recent Progression and Perspective

Kenichi Takayasu

Department of Diagnostic Radiology, National Cancer Center Hospital, Tokyo, Japan

Key Words
Hepatocellular carcinoma · Transcatheter arterial chemoembolization · Treatment algorithm · Japanese guidelines · BCLC staging system

Abstract
Transcatheter arterial chemoembolization (TACE) is widely performed in 32% of patients with unresectable hepatocellular carcinoma (HCC) at initial diagnosis and in 58% of those with recurrent HCC in Japan. However, the patient population which undergoes TACE is heterogeneous, and thus the 3-year survival rate varies from 26 to 47%. The selection criteria for TACE is 2–3 tumors >3 cm or 4 or more tumors in patients with liver damage A/B (corresponding well to Child-Pugh class A/B) and absence of vascular invasion and extrahepatic spread, as proposed by Japanese guidelines. The 3-year survival rate of TACE for patients with 2–3 tumors >3 cm or 4 or more tumors was 55 and 46%, respectively, in Child-Pugh A and 30 and 22%, respectively, in class B. These outcomes could help in understanding the various results of TACE in different backgrounds in the East and West. Recently, TACE with calibrated drug-eluting beads loaded with doxorubicin showed a similar tumor response and radioembolization with yttrium-90 microspheres demonstrated a similar median survival compared with conventional TACE. Based on these results, the combination of TACE and novel molecular targeted agents can be used to elucidate the synergic effect on survival.

Introduction

Hepatocellular carcinoma (HCC) is the 6th most common cancer and the 3rd leading cause of cancer-related death worldwide [1] and its incidence is increasing in Western countries [2, 3]. Curative treatments including resection, liver transplantation and local ablation are performed in only ~30% of patients, and transcatheter arterial chemoembolization (TACE) or sorafenib is used in ~50% of cases [4–6]. In Japan, resection is carried out in 32% of patients, local ablation in 31% and TACE including transcatheter arterial infusion chemotherapy in 32%, and other treatments [7]. For recurrent HCC, TACE is the mainstay treatment and is performed in 58% of patients.

Two randomized controlled trials (RCT) identified that TACE showed a significant survival benefit compared with controls [8, 9] after long-term controversy. Concerning the efficacy of TACE and transcatheter arterial embolization (TAE), one meta-analysis revealed a significant benefit of TACE with cisplatin or doxorubicin in 4 studies (n = 323, OR 0.42; 95% CI 0.20–0.88) but not with TAE alone in 3 studies (n = 215, OR 0.59; 95% CI 0.29–1.20) compared with controls [10]. However, they did not mention a direct superiority of TACE to TAE. Moreover, one systematic review showed no survival benefit of TACE over TAE in 3 RCTs (n = 412, OR 1.384; 95% CI 0.94–2.04); TAE appeared to be as effective as TACE [11].

KARGER

Fax +41 61 306 12 34
E-Mail karger@karger.com
www.karger.com

0030–2414/13/0847–0028$38.00/0

Accessible online at:
www.karger.com/ocl

Kenichi Takayasu
Department of Diagnostic Radiology
National Cancer Center Hospital
5-1-1 Tsukiji, Chuo-Ku, Tokyo 104-0045 (Japan)
E-Mail ktakayas@ncc.go.jp

To date, treatment algorithms for HCC have been proposed by the Barcelona Clinic Liver Cancer (BCLC) staging system [12–14] and by Japanese guidelines [15, 16]. For example, TACE is indicated in multinodular tumors (irrespective of size) in the intermediate stage of the BCLC, and 2–3 tumors >3 cm or 4 or more tumors in patients with degree of liver damage A/B and without macroscopic vascular invasion and extrahepatic spread in Japanese guidelines. The criteria for TACE seem to be very similar [17]. However, the survival rate of patients who undergo TACE and who fulfill the criteria determined by these two guidelines is still unclear.

Patients

Due to the nationwide prevalence of a surveillance system with periodical ultrasonography and alpha-fetoprotein measurement for at-risk patients, early-stage HCC could be detected with relative ease in Japan. Tumors ≤2 cm in diameter were found in 33.5% of patients, 57.7% had solitary tumors, 86.9% had no portal vein invasion and 71.0% were Child-Pugh class A [7]. Moreover, some 50% of patients are diagnosed in the intermediate or advanced stage in Western countries [4]. Recently, interesting news was reported that the detection rate of very early HCC had increased and the number of advanced tumors was reduced after the introduction of a semiannual surveillance system following an annual one [18].

Rationale and Procedure

The rationale for TACE is based on the dual supply of the liver, the hepatic artery and portal vein. The HCC is nourished by arterial blood flow and becomes ischemic and necrotic after embolization of the feeding artery, and noncancerous hepatic parenchyma survives due to a preserved portal blood supply. Generally, TACE is contraindicated in patients with Child-Pugh class C, macroscopic portal invasion or extrahepatic spread.

A great effort has been made to improve survival, to enhance the therapeutic effect of TACE on tumors and to lessen the adverse effects on noncancerous hepatic parenchyma. To achieve these goals, super-selective, subsegmental or targeted TACE was developed with a thin microcatheter system (2 or 3 Fr) and a mixture of anticancer agent and lipiodol followed by gelatin sponge particles [19–22]. Several imaging modalities such as a unified CT and angiography system [21] and recently CT-like images produced by C-arm digital subtraction angiography with a flat-panel detector [23] have facilitated the certainty and safety of super-selective embolization.

The usefulness of anticancer agents used in embolization is still controversial; one systematic review is against the use of anticancer agents [11] and another one seems to support it [10]. As of May 2006, the most common sole anticancer agent used worldwide was doxorubicin (36%), followed by cisplatin (31%) and epirubicin/doxorubicin (12%) [11]. Recently in Japan, epirubicin (69.0%) was chiefly used followed by doxorubicin (8.7%), mitomycin C (7.3%), zinostatin stimalamer (5.7%), cisplatin (5.2%) and others reported by the Liver Cancer Study Group of Japan (January 2004 to December 2005); this is mainly because epirubicin is covered by the National Insurance System but doxorubicin is not. More recently, a novel lipophilic cisplatin derivative has become commercially available; miriplatin hydrate, SM-11355 (*cis*-[((1R, 2R)-1, 2-cyclohexanediamine-N, N′) bis(myristato)]-platinum (II) monohydrate; Sumitomo Pharmaceutical Co., Osaka, Japan) compounds with lipiodol more easily and releases the drug gradually to tumor cells, resulting in minimization of the dose to flow in the systemic circulation [24].

Lipiodol is routinely used in TACE procedures in Japan where solitary HCCs up to 2 cm are very frequently found and treated using the technique of super-selective TACE if it is indicated. Lipiodol could obstruct thinner feeding arteries as well as accompanying portal veins through the peribiliary arterial plexus in which stasis is more tightly kept following the addition of embolization material. Moreover, a dose of lipiodol drains from the tumor via blood sinusoids to the peritumoral portal vessels, is histologically confirmed within fibrous capsules, and finally deposits in the noncancerous surrounding parenchyma [22, 25]. Thereby, infarction of the tumor as well as of the surrounding parenchyma occurs, which results in blockage of the development of new collateral arteries around the tumor. It is presumed that calibrated beads such as drug-eluting beads (DEB) and Embo-Sphere® available in Western countries do not show phenomena similar to those seen when lipiodol is used. Some beads are now being tested and compared with gelatin sponge plus lipiodol in Japan and the results are anticipated. The mean dose of lipiodol used by the LCSGJ in TACE was 5 ml (January 2004 to December 2005) [26]; which was much less than the median dose of lipiodol of 10 ml (range 2–25) reported by a systematic review [11].

Survival Rate

The median survival was 34 months, and the 1-, 2-, 3- and 5-year survival rates were 82, 63, 47 and 26% in 8,510 patients with unresectable HCC who underwent TACE with lipiodol during the last 8 years (January 1994 to December 2001) as reported by the LCSGJ [27]. According to a systematic analysis [11], Eastern trials showed better 3- and 5-year survival rates (33 ± 22 and 24 ± 14%, respectively) compared to Western ones (27 ± 9% and 7 ± 10%, respectively) in nonrandomized clinical studies. The 3-year survival rate of 47% in our study was above those in both Eastern and Western studies, whereas the 5-year survival rate of 26% was similar to the rate of 24 ± 14% found in Eastern studies. In two positive RCTs, the 3-year survival rate of TACE was 26 [9] and 29% [8].

Most nonrandomized clinical studies of TACE for unresectable HCC have heterogeneous populations, especially those conducted before 2000. Therefore, the survival rate of patients who fulfill the criteria of TACE for HCC is unclear. The 4,966 patients who were Child-Pugh A/B and received TACE were stratified into four treatment categories according to the treatment algorithm of Japanese guidelines. The patients stratified to TACE therapy for 2–3 tumors >3 cm or 4 or more tumors had a 3-year survival rate of 55 and 46% in the Child-Pugh A group; this was better than the rates of 30 and 22% found in class B [26]. The 3-year survival rate of 29% in one of the positive RCTs [8] appears to be comparable to the 30% found in our patients with 2–3 tumors >3 cm in Child-Pugh B. These outcomes might help in understanding the results of TACE in different backgrounds in the East and West and to design an RCT using TACE with and without novel molecular targeting agents.

Lewandowski et al. [28] reported the outcome of TACE with lipiodol in 172 patients with HCC; the overall median time to progression was 7.9 months and the median survival of patients in stages A, B and C of the BCLC staging system was 40.0, 17.4 and 6.3 months, respectively, with a significant difference. The median treatment-related 30-day mortality rate was 2.4% (range 0–9.5) as reported by a systematic review [11] and 0.5% as reported by the LCSGJ [27].

Prognostic Factors

Liver function, performance status, stage of cancer (number of tumors, tumor size, macroscopic vascular invasion and extrahepatic spread), alpha-fetoprotein, treatment, and skillfulness of the operator are prognostic factors of TACE for HCC [27, 29, 30]. The definition of repeated TACE is crucial, i.e. which method is adopted – on-demand based on the tumor response or new recurrence on follow-up images or set interval. Multiple sessions of TACE frequently induce vascular injury and hepatic atrophy. There is no prospective study comparing the survival benefits of these two different methods.

Drug-Eluting Beads

Novel embolization material of DEB loaded with doxorubicin has been developed [31]. Lammer et al. [32] conducted a randomized, single-blind, phase II study in HCC patients with Child-Pugh A/B status and evaluated the toxicity and tumor response of DEB-TACE loaded with doxorubicin (150 mg, n = 93 patients) compared with conventional TACE using an emulsion of doxorubicin (50–75 mg/m^2 to a maximum of 150 mg) and lipiodol followed by particle embolization (n = 108) at 6 months after the 2-month set interval. There was no significant difference between the two treatments. The subgroup analysis of more advanced patients with Child-Pugh B, bilobar disease and recurrent disease showed a significant increase in objective response compared with conventional TACE. DEB-TACE demonstrated a significantly lower serious liver toxicity and a lower rate of doxorubicin-related side effects such as alopecia and skin discoloration. The treatment-related 30-day mortality was 2 patients (2.2%) in DEB-TACE and 6 (5.6%) in conventional TACE. Thereafter, a comparative study of doxorubicin-eluted DEB and bland embolization using BeadBlock™ of the same size showed that DEB-TACE presented a better local response and a longer time to progression than bland embolization [33].

Radioembolization

Radioembolization with yttrium-90 (^{90}Y) microspheres emitting beta particles with a 64.1-hour physical half-life injected through the hepatic artery for HCC has been developed. Two ^{90}Y microsphere devices are commercially available: TheraSphere® (made of glass; MDS Nordion, Ottawa, Ont., Canada) and SIR-Spheres® (made of resin; Sirtex Medical, Sydney, N.S.W., Australia). Unlike external-beam radiation of one lobe or the entire liver, which frequently causes radiation-induced hepatitis, ^{90}Y radioembolization is internal radiation which emits high-energy and low-penetration radiation to tumors and the embolization effect is minimal. This property makes radioembolization possible for treating HCC associated with branch or lobar portal vein thrombosis (PVT) [34]; conventional TACE is relatively contraindicated in the latter. A side effect of this therapy is that ^{90}Y microspheres are delivered to the lung via the hepatopulmonary shunt seen in cirrhosis and to the gastrointestinal tract, resulting in serious complications such as gastric ulceration, gastroduodenitis, cholecystitis, pancreatitis and radiation pneumonitis.

Recently, a prospective cohort study of HCC with ^{90}Y radioembolization demonstrated that Child-Pugh A patients had a significantly better median survival time than did class B patients (17.2 vs. 7.7 months, respectively) [35]. Moreover, patients with PVT showed lower median survivals compared to those without it in both Child-Pugh A and B patients (class A, 10.4 vs. 22.1 months; class B, 5.6 vs. 14.8 months, respectively). They concluded that Child-Pugh A patients with or without PVT benefitted from ^{90}Y radioembolization and class B patients with PVT had a poor prognosis. The treatment-related 30-day mortality rate was 3%. Most recently, for 246 HCC patients without vascular invasion or extrahepatic spread, a comparative study of ^{90}Y radioembolization (1 session) and chemoembolization (median, 2 sessions) was performed. As a result, there was no significant difference in median overall survival between radioembolization and TACE (20.5 vs. 17.4 months, respectively, and in patients in the intermediate stage of the BCLC staging system, 17.2 vs. 17.5 months, respectively) [36]. Radioembolization showed a higher tumor response rate compared to chemoembolization (49 vs. 36%, $p = 0.104$).

Combination of TACE and Molecular Targeted Agents

Among several molecular targeted agents, sorafenib is a multikinase inhibitor with antiangiogenic and antiproliferative properties that targets multiple pathways [37, 38]. Two large randomized phase III studies demonstrated that sorafenib significantly prolongs overall survival in patients with advanced HCC [39, 40]. It is well known that ischemic or hypoxic changes of HCC after TACE/TAE induce an increase of vascular endothelial growth factor (VEGF) expression in the residual surviving cancerous tissue [41] and enhance the serum concentration of VEGF [42]. In a rabbit study, expression of hypoxia-inducible factor-1α in the nuclei of residual viable HCC cells after TAE was demonstrated [43]; it regulates the release of multiple angiogenic factors such as VEGF, basic fibroblast growth factor and insulin-like growth factor [44]. These results suggest that sorafenib may exert anti-angiogenic effects immediately or before TACE [45–47]. Several trials studying the combination of TACE and sorafenib or placebo are ongoing [DEB-TACE with 150 mg doxorubicin and sorafenib [48], and conventional TACE and sorafenib [49] or other agents of TSU-68 (orantinib)] [50]. A global RCT is underway and will be conducted with various combinations of established therapies such as TACE, resection, local ablation and new molecular targeted agents as well as cytotoxic agents, and a drastic paradigm shift in treatment is expected to occur.

Disclosure Statement

The author has no conflicts of interest to report.

References

1 Parkin DM, Bray F, Ferlay J, Pisani P: Global cancer statistics, 2002. CA Cancer J Clin 2005;55:74–108.
2 El-Serag HB: Hepatocellular carcinoma: recent trends in the United States. Gastroenterology 2004;127(5 suppl 1):S27–S34.
3 Fattovich G, Stroffolini T, Zagni I, Donato F. Hepatocellular carcinoma in cirrhosis: incidence and risk factors. Gastroenterology 2004;127(5 suppl 1):S35–S50.
4 Llovet JM, Di Bisceglie AM, Bruix J, Kramer BS, Lencioni R, Zhu AX, et al: Design and endpoints of clinical trials in hepatocellular carcinoma. J Natl Cancer Inst 2008;100:698–711.
5 Lencioni R: Chemoembolization in patients with hepatocellular carcinoma. Liver Cancer 2012;1:41–50.
6 Kudo M: Treatment of advanced hepatocellular carcinoma with emphasis on hepatic arterial infusion chemotherapy and molecular targeted therapy. Liver Cancer 2012;1:62–70.
7 Ikai I, Kudo M, Arii S, Omata M, Kojiro M, Sakamoto M, et al: Report of the 18th Nationwide Follow-Up Survey of Primary Liver Cancer in Japan. Hepatol Res 2010;40:1043–1059.
8 Llovet JM, Real MI, Montana X, Planas R, Coll S, Aponte J, et al: Arterial embolisation or chemoembolisation versus symptomatic treatment in patients with unresectable hepatocellular carcinoma: a randomised controlled trial. Lancet 2002;359:1734–1739.
9 Lo CM, Ngan H, Tso WK, Liu CL, Lam CM, Poon RT, et al: Randomized controlled trial of transarterial lipiodol chemoembolization for unresectable hepatocellular carcinoma. Hepatology 2002;35:1164–1171.
10 Llovet JM, Bruix J: Systematic review of randomized trials for unresectable hepatocellular carcinoma: chemoembolization improves survival. Hepatology 2003;37:429–442.

11 Marelli L, Stigliano R, Triantos C, Senzolo M, Cholongitas E, Davies N, et al: Transarterial therapy for hepatocellular carcinoma: which technique is more effective? A systematic review of cohort and randomized studies. Cardiovasc Intervent Radiol 2007;30:6–25.
12 Llovet JM, Bru C, Bruix J: Prognosis of hepatocellular carcinoma: the BCLC staging classification. Semin Liver Dis 1999;19:329–338.
13 Bruix J, Sherman M: Management of hepatocellular carcinoma. Hepatology 2005;42:1208–1236.
14 Lin S, Hoffmann K, Schemmer P: Treatment of hepatocellular carcinoma: a systematic review. Liver Cancer, in press.
15 Makuuchi M, Kokudo N, Arii S, Futagawa S, Kaneko S, Kawasaki S, et al: Development of evidence-based clinical guidelines for the diagnosis and treatment of hepatocellular carcinoma in Japan. Hepatol Res 2008;38:37–51.
16 Kudo M, Okanoue T: Management of hepatocellular carcinoma in Japan: consensus-based clinical practice manual proposed by the Japan Society of Hepatology. Oncology 2007;72(suppl 1):2–15.
17 Takayama T: Hepatocellular carcinoma; in Clavien PA (ed): Malignant Liver Tumors: Current and Emerging Therapies, ed 3. London, Wiley-Blackwell, 2010, pp 317–323.
18 Santi V, Trevisani F, Gramenzi A, Grignaschi A, Mirici-Cappa F, Poggio PD, et al: Semiannual surveillance is superior to annual surveillance for the detection of early hepatocellular carcinoma and patient survival. J Hepatol 2010;53:291–297.
19 Uchida H, Ohishi H, Matsuo N, Nishimine K, Ohue S, Nishimura Y, et al: Transcatheter hepatic segmental arterial embolization using lipiodol mixed with an anticancer drug and Gelfoam particles for hepatocellular carcinoma. Cardiovasc Intervent Radiol 1990;13:140–145.
20 Matsui O, Kadoya M, Yoshikawa J, Gabata T, Arai K, Demachi H, et al: Small hepatocellular carcinoma: treatment with subsegmental transcatheter arterial embolization. Radiology 1993;188:79–83.
21 Takayasu K, Muramatsu Y, Maeda T, Iwata R, Furukawa H, Moriyama N, et al: Targeted transarterial oily chemoembolization for small foci of hepatocellular carcinoma using a unified helical CT and angiography system: analysis of factors affecting local recurrence and survival rates. AJR Am J Roentgenol 2001;176:681–688.
22 Miyayama S, Matsui O, Yamashiro M, Ryu Y, Kaito K, Ozaki K, et al: Ultraselective transcatheter arterial chemoembolization with a 2-f tip microcatheter for small hepatocellular carcinomas: relationship between local tumor recurrence and visualization of the portal vein with iodized oil. J Vasc Interv Radiol 2007;18:365–376.
23 Iwazawa J, Ohue S, Mitani T, Abe H, Hashimoto N, Hamuro M, et al: Identifying feeding arteries during TACE of hepatic tumors: comparison of C-arm CT and digital subtraction angiography. AJR Am J Roentgenol 2009;192:1057–1063.
24 Okusaka T, Okada S, Nakanishi T, Fujiyama S, Kubo Y: Phase II trial of intra-arterial chemotherapy using a novel lipophilic platinum derivative (SM-11355) in patients with hepatocellular carcinoma. Invest New Drugs 2004;22:169–176.
25 Terayama N, Matsui O, Gabata T, Kobayashi S, Sanada J, Ueda K, et al: Accumulation of iodized oil within the nonneoplastic liver adjacent to hepatocellular carcinoma via the drainage routes of the tumor after transcatheter arterial embolization. Cardiovasc Intervent Radiol 2001;24:383–387.
26 Takayasu K, Arii S, Kudo M, Ichida T, Matsui O, Izumi N, et al: Superselective transarterial chemoembolization for hepatocellular carcinoma: validation of treatment algorithm proposed by Japanese guidelines. J Hepatol 2012;56:886–892.
27 Takayasu K, Arii S, Ikai I, Omata M, Okita K, Ichida T, et al: Prospective cohort study of transarterial chemoembolization for unresectable hepatocellular carcinoma in 8,510 patients. Gastroenterology 2006;131:461–469.
28 Lewandowski RJ, Mulcahy MF, Kulik LM, Riaz A, Ryu RK, Baker TB, et al: Chemoembolization for hepatocellular carcinoma: comprehensive imaging and survival analysis in a 172-patient cohort. Radiology 2010;255:955–965.
29 Ueno K, Miyazono N, Inoue H, Nishida H, Kanetsuki I, Nakajo M: Transcatheter arterial chemoembolization therapy using iodized oil for patients with unresectable hepatocellular carcinoma: evaluation of three kinds of regimens and analysis of prognostic factors. Cancer 2000;88:1574–1581.
30 Raoul JL, Sangro B, Forner A, Mazzaferro V, Piscaglia F, Bolondi L, et al: Evolving strategies for the management of intermediate-stage hepatocellular carcinoma: available evidence and expert opinion on the use of transarterial chemoembolization. Cancer Treat Rev 2011;37:212–220.
31 Varela M, Real MI, Burrel M, Forner A, Sala M, Brunet M, et al: Chemoembolization of hepatocellular carcinoma with drug eluting beads: efficacy and doxorubicin pharmacokinetics. J Hepatol 2007;46:474–481.
32 Lammer J, Malagari K, Vogl T, Pilleul F, Denys A, Watkinson A, et al: Prospective randomized study of doxorubicin-eluting-bead embolization in the treatment of hepatocellular carcinoma: results of the PRECISION V study. Cardiovasc Intervent Radiol 2010;33:41–52.
33 Malagari K, Pomoni M, Kelekis A, Pomoni A, Dourakis S, Spyridopoulos T, et al: Prospective randomized comparison of chemoembolization with doxorubicin-eluting beads and bland embolization with BeadBlock for hepatocellular carcinoma. Cardiovasc Intervent Radiol 2010;33:541–551.
34 Kulik LM, Carr BI, Mulcahy MF, Lewandowski RJ, Atassi B, Ryu RK, et al: Safety and efficacy of 90Y radiotherapy for hepatocellular carcinoma with and without portal vein thrombosis. Hepatology 2008;47:71–81.
35 Salem R, Lewandowski RJ, Mulcahy MF, Riaz A, Ryu RK, Ibrahim S, et al: Radioembolization for hepatocellular carcinoma using yttrium-90 microspheres: a comprehensive report of long-term outcomes. Gastroenterology 2010;138:52–64.
36 Salem R, Lewandowski RJ, Kulik L, Wang E, Riaz A, Ryu RK, et al: Radioembolization results in longer time-to-progression and reduced toxicity compared with chemoembolization in patients with hepatocellular carcinoma. Gastroenterology 2011;140:497–507.
37 Wilhelm SM, Carter C, Tang L, Wilkie D, McNabola A, Rong H, et al: BAY 43-9006 exhibits broad spectrum oral antitumor activity and targets the RAF/MEK/ERK pathway and receptor tyrosine kinases involved in tumor progression and angiogenesis. Cancer Res 2004;64:7099–7109.
38 Carlomagno F, Anaganti S, Guida T, Salvatore G, Troncone G, Wilhelm SM, et al: BAY 43-9006 inhibition of oncogenic RET mutants. J Natl Cancer Inst 2006;98:326–334.
39 Llovet JM, Ricci S, Mazzaferro V, Hilgard P, Gane E, Blanc JF, et al: Sorafenib in advanced hepatocellular carcinoma. N Engl J Med 2008;359:378–390.
40 Cheng AL, Kang YK, Chen Z, Tsao CJ, Qin S, Kim JS, et al: Efficacy and safety of sorafenib in patients in the Asia-Pacific region with advanced hepatocellular carcinoma: a phase III randomised, double-blind, placebo-controlled trial. Lancet Oncol 2009;10:25–34.
41 Wang B, Xu H, Gao ZQ, Ning HF, Sun YQ, Cao GW: Increased expression of vascular endothelial growth factor in hepatocellular carcinoma after transcatheter arterial chemoembolization. Acta Radiol 2008;49:523–529.
42 Li X, Feng GS, Zheng CS, Zhuo CK, Liu X: Expression of plasma vascular endothelial growth factor in patients with hepatocellular carcinoma and effect of transcatheter arterial chemoembolization therapy on plasma vascular endothelial growth factor level. World J Gastroenterol 2004;10:2878–2882.
43 Virmani S, Rhee TK, Ryu RK, Sato KT, Lewandowski RJ, Mulcahy MF, et al: Comparison of hypoxia-inducible factor-1α expression before and after transcatheter arterial embolization in rabbit VX2 liver tumors. J Vasc Interv Radiol 2008;19:1483–1489.

44 Sun HC, Tang ZY: Angiogenesis in hepatocellular carcinoma: the retrospectives and perspectives. J Cancer Res Clin Oncol 2004; 130:307–319.
45 Kudo M, Imanaka K, Chida N, Nakachi K, Tak WY, Takayama T, et al: Phase III study of sorafenib after transarterial chemoembolisation in Japanese and Korean patients with unresectable hepatocellular carcinoma. Eur J Cancer 2011;47:2117–2127.
46 Hsu C, Liang PC, Morita S, Hu FC, Cheng AL: Perspectives on the design of clinical trials combining transarterial chemoembolization and molecular targeted therapy. Liver Cancer, in press.
47 Liapi E, Geschwind JF: Combination of local transcatheter arterial chemoembolization and systemic anti-angiogenic therapy for unresectable hepatocellular carcinoma. Liver Cancer, in press.
48 Lencioni R, Zou J, Leberre M, Meinhardt G, Voliotis D, Bruix J, et al: Sorafenib (SOR) or placebo (PL) in combination with transarterial chemoembolization (TACE) for intermediate-stage hepatocellular carcinoma (SPACE). J Clin Oncol 2010;28(suppl): abstr TPS178).
49 Chung Y, Kim B, Chen C, Wang J, Chu H, Yoon J, et al: Study in Asia of the combination of transcatheter arterial chemoembolization (TACE) with sorafenib in patients with hepatocellular carcinoma (HCC) trial (START): second interim safety and efficacy analysis. J Clin Oncol 2010;28(suppl): abstr 4026.
50 Arai Y, Inaba Y, Yamamoto T, Kanai F, Aramaki T, et al: A randomized phase II study of TSU-68 in patients (pts) with hepatocellular carcinoma (HCC) treated by transarterial chemoembolization (TACE). J Clin Oncol 2010;28(suppl): abstr 4030.

Oncology

Oncology 2013;84(suppl 1):34–39
DOI: 10.1159/000345887

Published online: February 20, 2013

Yttrium-90 Radioembolization for Hepatocellular Carcinoma: What We Know and What We Need to Know

Yun Hwan Kim[a] Do Young Kim[b]

[a]Department of Radiology, Korea University College of Medicine, and [b]Department of Internal Medicine, Yonsei University College of Medicine, Seoul, Korea

Key Words

Hepatocellular carcinoma · Yttrium-90 · Transarterial chemoembolization

Abstract

In spite of substantial progress in the management of hepatocellular carcinoma (HCC), suboptimal treatment results are frequently seen in the intermediate and advanced stages of HCC. The current staging system indicates that multinodular HCC without vascular invasion needs to be treated by transarterial chemoembolization (TACE) and HCC with vascular nvasion or distant metastasis is linked to sorafenib, an antiangiogenic therapy. Radioembolization with yttrium-90 (^{90}Y) is a recently introduced liver-directed therapy employing a catheter-based approach. Growing data suggest that ^{90}Y radioembolization has a potent anticancer effect with negligible adverse events if appropriate pretreatment evaluations including dosimetry, calculation of lung shunt fraction and assessment of vascular anatomy are performed. Retrospective and small prospective studies have shown response rates and survival after ^{90}Y therapy which are comparable to TACE and sorafenib in the intermediate and advanced stages, respectively. Although a large sample size is necessary to compare the outcome between TACE and radioembolization in intermediate-stage HCC, selected populations, for whom TACE would not be effective, are candidates for testing the role of ^{90}Y radioembolization. A multidisciplinary, combined approach in advanced HCC using loco-regional therapy such as radioembolization and systemic therapy including sorafenib also has to be investigated.

Introduction

Despite substantial progress in diagnosis and treatment, hepatocellular carcinoma (HCC) is a difficult disease to cure, particularly when it presents in an advanced stage [1]. The current popular staging system, the Barcelona Clinic Liver Cancer (BCLC) stage, indicates that multinodular HCC without vascular invasion (BCLC-B stage) is linked to transarterial chemoembolization (TACE) [2], whereas systemic therapy might be beneficial in HCC with distant metastasis or vascular invasion (BCLC-C) [3]. Although accumulated data suggest that TACE could increase survival of patients with unresectable HCC [4], the efficacy of this modality in cases with large size or multiple tumors is not satisfactory [5]. Sorafenib, a receptor tyrosine kinase inhibitor, opened the window for targeted therapy in the management of HCC and has been accepted for use in advanced HCC such as extrahepatic metastasis or portal vein invasion [6–8]. However, prolongation of time to

KARGER

Fax +41 61 306 12 34
E-Mail karger@karger.com
www.karger.com

0030–2414/13/0847–0034$38.00/0

Accessible online at:
www.karger.com/ocl

Yun Hwan Kim, MD
Department of Radiology, Anam Hospital, Korea University College of Medicine
126-1, 5-Ka, Anam-Dong, Sungbuk-Gu
Seoul 136-705 (Korea)
E-Mail yhkku@kumc.or.kr

progression or overall survival was found to be marginal in hepatitis B virus-associated HCC, which is predominant, especially in Asia, including Korea [9]. In this regards, another breakthrough is definitely needed for the optimal management of intermediate- to advanced-stage HCC.

Yttrium-90 (^{90}Y) radioembolization is an emerging catheter-based therapy in which the source of radiation accesses the network of tumoral vessels after being injected into the hepatic arteries. Microspheres made of resin (SIR-Spheres®; Sirtex Medical, Sidney, N.S.W., Australia) or glass (TheraSphere®, MDS Nordion, Toronto, Ont., Canada) are loaded with ^{90}Y to allow distribution of radioisotopes through tumor-feeding arteries. ^{90}Y is a pure beta-emitter, and generates high-energy radiation with a short half-life (2.67 days), and a short tissue penetration (mean 2.5 mm, maximum 11 mm) [10].

Available data tell us that ^{90}Y radioembolization could be an option for intermediate- to advanced-stage HCC. Here, we intend to summarize the recent results of ^{90}Y radioembolization regarding treatment response, survival, adverse event and appropriate indication as well as unsolved issues.

Technical Aspect

Prior to the procedure of radioembolization, all patients should receive a test using ^{99m}Tc-labeled macroaggregated albumin to see whether the pulmonary shunt is less than 20% or not. If the fraction of pulmonary shunt is greater than 20%, the systemic distribution of radioactive isotope and resulting toxicity are anticipated. Any uncorrectable delivery of ^{90}Y to the gastrointestinal tract, reverse blood flow out of the liver, or complete portal vein thrombosis are contraindications of radioembolization and the presence of these is also evaluated together with shunt study by preangiography before treatment [11]. If necessary, embolizing of nontarget vessels is performed to minimize the flow of ^{90}Y microspheres into both uninvolved liver parenchyma and extrahepatic tissues.

Estimation of the radiation dose actually delivered to tumor tissue is complicated. The basic premise for ^{90}Y microsphere dosimetry is to ensure that the liver parenchyma exposure does not exceed 70 Gy, while at least 120 Gy must accumulate within the tumor to deliver a dose-dependent tumoricidal effect [12]. Accurate assessment of target tumor and liver volume is critical because it directly affects radiation absorbed dose estimates. The desired ^{90}Y activity is calculated using a partition model or body surface area model [13]. Infusion of the microspheres into one or both lobes can generally be accomplished in a single session unless the patient has impaired liver function, in which case two procedures separated by 30–45 days might be required [14]. Unlike TACE, it is recommended that assessment of response to radioembolization needs to be done at approximately 3 months postprocedure due to the delayed radiation effect on the tumor [15].

Response to ^{90}Y Radioembolization

Due to the heterogeneous populations recruited and the time point of assessment, the reported response rates to ^{90}Y radioembolization are variable among studies published so far. Partial response representing a 51–87% reduction in tumor volume was observed in 26.7% of the initial experience of this modality [16].

In a European prospective study of 52 patients with median follow-up of 36 months, 5 complete responses (9.6%) occurred. The objective response and disease control rate were 40.4 and 78.8%, respectively, when European Association for the Study of the Liver (EASL) criteria was applied for the assessment of tumor response [17]. A retrospective study of 123 patients who had been treated by ^{90}Y radioembolization in the USA reported that overall response measured by EASL criteria was observed in 88 (72%) patients compared with 69% in those who received TACE ($p = 0.748$) [18]. ^{90}Y radioembolization was performed in a total of 108 consecutive HCC patients in a German multicenter study, of whom 76 patients were available for assessment of treatment response. With EASL criteria, complete response was achieved in 2 (3%) patients, partial response in 23 (37%) and stable disease in 33 (53%) patients at 3 months post-treatment [19]. The efficacy of ^{90}Y radioembolization in HCC with portal vein invasion is controversial. In a retrospective study of 22 patients with main (n = 10) or first-branch (n = 12) portal vein invasion, the partial response rate was 8%, stable disease was achieved in 50% and progressive disease was seen in 42% [20]. A large-series of cohort studies in which 291 patients were treated with ^{90}Y reported that overall response rates based on EASL criteria were 57% [21].

Survival and Prognostic Factors

In 71 patients including 20 patients with postoperative recurrence, the median survival was 9.4 months (range 1.8–46.4) [16]. In a series of 325 patients recruited from

Table 1. A summary of response rates, survival and prognostic factors after ^{90}Y treatment from recent studies

Author, year	n	Response rate	Survival	Prognostic factors
Mazzaferro, 2012 [17]	52	CR 9.6%; OR 40.4%	15 months	Response; Child-Pugh score
Sangro, 2012 [29]	325		12.8 months	ECOG status; nodules >5; INR >1.2; extrahepatic disease
Salem, 2011 [18]	123	RR 72%	20.5 months	Female sex; Child-Pugh class; UNOS stage
Kulik, 2008 [35]	71	PR 42%; SD 35%	15.5 months	
Young, 2007 [38]	41		Okuda I: 21.7 months Okuda II: 14.2 months	
Sangro, 2006 [39]	24	PR 24%; SD 64%	7 months	
Salem, 2005 [23]	43	PR 47%	Okuda I: 24 months Okuda II: 13 months	Main PVT; AFP >400 ng/ml; >25% tumor burden
Carr, 2004 [40]	65	OR 38%	Okuda I: 21 months Okuda II: 10 months	

AFP = Alpha-fetoprotein; CR = complete response; RR = response rate; OR = objective response; PR = partial response; SD = stable disease; ECOG = European Cooperative Oncology Group; PVT = portal vein thrombosis; UNOS = the United Network of Organ Sharing.

European multicenters, over half had BCLC-C staging (56.3%) and a quarter had BCLC-B staging (26.8%). The median overall survival was 12.8 months (95% CI 10.9–15.7). The median survival in BCLC-A, B and C was 24.4 months (95% CI 18.6–38.1), 16.9 months (95% CI 12.8–2.8), and 10.0 months (95% CI 7.7–10.9), respectively. In another European study with a small number of patients (n = 52), median overall survival was not significantly different between HCC with portal vein thrombosis and HCC without (18 vs. 13 months), suggesting the role of ^{90}Y therapy in the management of HCC with vascular invasion [17]. However, in a study of 291 patients from the USA, patients with Child-Pugh B who also had portal vein thrombosis just survived 5.6 months (95% CI 4.5–6.7) [21]. The predictors of survival are not consistent among studies, although initial response to radioembolization might be one of the most important prognostic indicators [17, 21]. Table 1 summarizes the response rate, survival and prognostic factors in the recent studies.

Safety of ^{90}Y Radioembolization

The major concern regarding ^{90}Y therapy comes from the recognition that radioactive substance is injected into human body. However, serious adverse events related to radiation can be avoided if proper patients are selected, accepted dosimetry models are used and meticulous technique is employed [22]. Postradioembolization syndrome consists of fatigue, nausea, vomiting, anorexia, fever and abdominal pain. The incidence of this ranges from 20 to 55% [23, 24], and the degree of symptoms is reported to be less severe than so-called postembolization syndrome observed after conventional TACE [25]. Radiation-induced liver disease is characterized by deterioration of liver function and the incidence is reported to range from 0 to 4% depending on the preexisting liver function abnormality [26]. In case of spillage of microspheres into cystic artery, radiation-induced cholecystitis may occur. Other biliary sequelae include biliary necrosis, biloma, liver abscess and biliary strictures [27]. The information from the pretreatment angiography can minimize gastrointestinal complications after ^{90}Y therapy. Careful dose adjustment of yttrium to prevent nontumoral parenchymal damage, resulting hepatic volume contraction and portal hypertension is required. Monitoring of development of radiation pneumonitis is necessary if lung shunt fraction is greater than 13% [28].

^{90}Y Therapy versus TACE in Intermediate-Stage HCC

Although survival after radioembolization has been reported to be promising for those patients that are ideal candidates for TACE, with median overall survival of 22.8 months (95% CI 13.6–36.0) for patients with 1–5 nodules and 23.2 months for tumors affecting a single lobe [29], there are not sufficient data prospectively comparing the efficacy in terms of response or survival between radioembolization and TACE in the intermediate

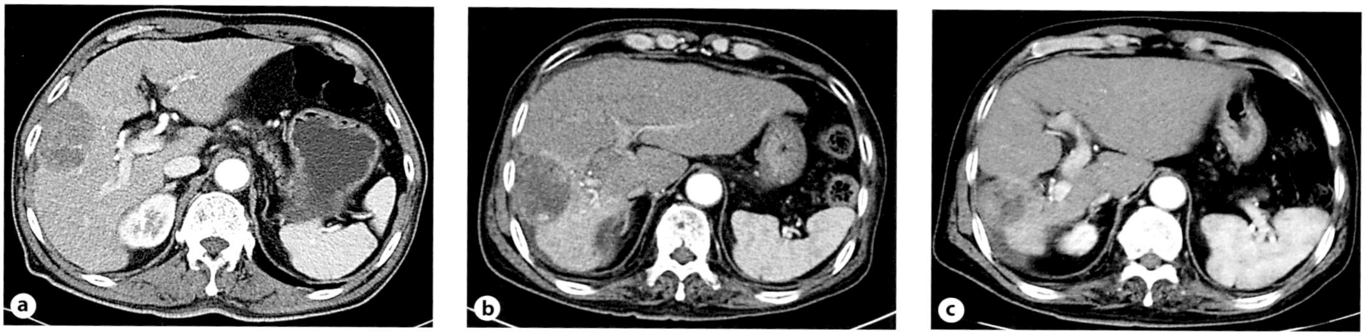

Fig. 1. a Pretreatment arterial phase CT scan. A 6-cm, hypervascular round HCC is seen in the right lobe of the liver. **b** One-year post-^{90}Y radioembolization CT scan. Arterial enhancement is still seen inside the HCC. Arterial-portal shunt posterior to the mass, right lobe atrophy and compensatory left lobe hypertrophy are also noticed. **c**. Three-year post-^{90}Y therapy CT scan (arterial phase). The tumor has shrunk, however, a faint hypervascularity is still observed inside the tumor.

stage. Indeed, growing evidence suggests that over 1,000 patients would be required to demonstrate the difference of survival between these two modalities [18]. In a retrospective study comparing the outcomes between radioembolization (n = 38) and TACE (n = 35), there was no significant difference in survival (median 8.0 vs. 10.3 months, p = 0.33), although postembolization syndrome was significantly more severe in patients who underwent chemoembolization [30]. In another retrospective study, patients with BCLC-B exhibited nearly identical survival times (17.5 vs. 17.2 months, p = 0.42) between ^{90}Y therapy and TACE [18]. It might be highlighted that the BCLC-B stage includes various tumor characteristics in terms of tumor number and size. TACE cannot lead to effective tumor control for large tumor with multiple satellite nodules, instead, patients with these tumor characteristics usually experience severe postembolization syndrome. Thus, comparing the efficacy and safety between ^{90}Y and TACE focusing on large HCCs would be necessary. Obviously, it is also required to assess the cost-effectiveness of radioembolization in intermediate-stage HCC, considering whether the high cost of ^{90}Y can balance the long hospital stay due to complications and the cumulating charge of repeated TACE, especially in Asian countries.

^{90}Y Therapy in Advanced Stage

Most international liver societies guide HCC with vascular invasion or distant metastasis to treatment with sorafenib, a proven molecular targeted agent [3, 31–33]. For HCC with vascular invasion, any treatment other than sorafenib has not been shown to be effective in prolonging patient survival compared with supportive care. In a pilot study, external radiation therapy for HCC with portal vein thrombosis was shown to result in a promising outcome. Of 40 patients who underwent concurrent regional chemotherapy using intra-arterial implanted port plus localized external beam radiotherapy of 45 Gy over 5 weeks, the 3-year overall survival rate was 24.1% and the median time was 13.1 months [34]. As for ^{90}Y radioembolization for advanced HCC, only limited data are currently available. Unlike external beam radiation therapy where main portal vein thrombosis is not a contraindication, total occlusion of the vessel may increase the risk of hepatic decompensation after radioembolization. In a phase II trial, the median survival of patients with branch portal vein thrombosis after ^{90}Y was 261 days, while that of patients with main portal vein thrombosis was 148 days [35]. Due to lack of a well-designed randomized study, it is hard to compare the efficacy of ^{90}Y therapy in HCC with advanced stage compared with sorafenib, though a few series have reported that the median overall survival of patients treated with ^{90}Y was either comparable to even higher than that of sorafenib treatment [19, 21]. The result of an ongoing trial prospectively comparing radioembolization and sorafenib in advanced-stage HCC will tell us more about the position of ^{90}Y therapy in HCC management.

Uncertainty Regarding ^{90}Y Therapy

Figure 1 shows the case of a 71-year-old male HCC patient who underwent ^{90}Y radioembolization in July 2009. The baseline serum alpha-fetoprotein (AFP) levels were 45.8 ng/ml. After one session of ^{90}Y therapy had been performed, hypervascularity within the tumor was still seen on follow-up CT scan taken 1 year later (July 2010) and the serum AFP level was 29.7 ng/ml. Without more treatment, the arterial enhancing portion was even observed 3 years later (July 2012), although the size of HCC was reduced (serum AFP = 13.4 ng/ml). In this patient, des-γ-prothrombin was not helpful for monitoring after ^{90}Y therapy since warfarin was administered due to an old cerebrovascular accident. There are not sufficient data to guide additional therapy for remnant arterial enhancing lesion within ^{90}Y-treated mass, especially when tumor marker such as AFP or des-γ-prothrombin level is not increased. As with other treatment modalities, pretherapy imaging or biomarker predictors of response or survival need to be found. As previously pointed out, the spatial distribution of the microspheres is very irregular, and the resulting dose distribution is highly heterogeneous, which could induce the risk of small cold spots inside tumor tissue [36, 37]. The usefulness of combined treatment with ^{90}Y radioembolization and sorafenib or other systemic therapy in HCC with vascular invasion and extrahepatic metastasis has to be investigated.

Conclusion

Intermediate- and advanced-stage HCC remain challenging to physicians and interventional radiologists because of suboptimal tumor control and frequent relapse even after induction of complete tumor necrosis by a catheter-based approach. A potent anticancer effect given by ^{90}Y administered through the hepatic arteries might be a good opportunity to complement therapeutic modalities utilized so far. Further investigations about the cost-effectiveness of ^{90}Y radioembolization and determination of appropriate indications are necessary.

Disclosure Statement

No financial disclosures reported.

References

1 Kudo M: Japan's successful model of nationwide hepatocellular carcinoma surveillance highlighting the urgent need for global surveillance. Liver Cancer, in press.
2 Lencioni R: Chemoembolization in patients with hepatocellular carcinoma. Liver Cancer 2012;1:41–50.
3 Llovet JM, Ducreux M, Lencioni R, et al: EASL-EORTC clinical practice guidelines: management of hepatocellular carcinoma. J Hepatol 2012;56:908–943.
4 Llovet JM, Bruix J: Systematic review of randomized trials for unresectable hepatocellular carcinoma: chemoembolization improves survival. Hepatology 2003;37:429–442.
5 Kim DY, Ryu HJ, Choi JY, Park JY, Lee DY, Kim BK, Kim SU, Ahn SH, Chon CY, Han KH: Radiological response predicts survival following transarterial chemoembolisation in patients with unresectable hepatocellular carcinoma. Aliment Pharmacol Ther 2012;35:1343–1350.
6 Llovet JM, Ricci S, Mazzaferro V, Hilgard P, Gane E, Blanc JF, de Oliveira AC, Santoro A, Raoul JL, Forner A, Schwartz M, Porta C, Zeuzem S, Bolondi L, Greten TF, Galle PR, Seitz JF, Borbath I, Haussinger D, Giannaris T, Shan M, Moscovici M, Voliotis D, Bruix J: Sorafenib in advanced hepatocellular carcinoma. N Engl J Med 2008;359:378–390.
7 Kudo M: Treatment of advanced hepatocellular carcinoma with emphasis on hepatic arterial infusion chemotherapy and molecular targeted therapy. Liver Cancer 2012;1:62–70.
8 Choi GH, Shim JH, Lee D, Kim KM, Ryu MH, Lim YS, Ryoo BY, Lee HC, Chung YH, Kang YK, Lee YS, Suh DJ: The optimal indication of sorafenib treatment in patients with advanced-stage hepatocellular carcinoma. Liver Cancer 2012;1:115.
9 Bruix J, Raoul JL, Sherman M, Mazzaferro V, Bolondi L, Craxi A, Galle PR, Santoro A, Beaugrand M, Sangiovanni A, Porta C, Gerken G, Marrero JA, Nadel A, Shan M, Moscovici M, Voliotis D, Llovet JM: Efficacy and safety of sorafenib in patients with advanced hepatocellular carcinoma: subanalyses of a phase III trial. J Hepatol 2012;57:821–829.
10 Sangro B, Inarrairaegui M, Bilbao JI: Radioembolization for hepatocellular carcinoma. J Hepatol 2012;56:464–473.
11 Strigari L, Sciuto R, Rea S, Carpanese L, Pizzi G, Soriani A, Iaccarino G, Benassi M, Ettorre GM, Maini CL: Efficacy and toxicity related to treatment of hepatocellular carcinoma with ^{90}Y-SIR spheres: radiobiologic considerations. J Nucl Med 2010;51:1377–1385.
12 Ho S, Lau WY, Leung TW, Chan M, Johnson PJ, Li AK: Clinical evaluation of the partition model for estimating radiation doses from yttrium-90 microspheres in the treatment of hepatic cancer. Eur J Nucl Med 1997;24:293–298.
13 Kao YH, Tan EH, Ng CE, Goh SW: Clinical implications of the body surface area method versus partition model dosimetry for yttrium-90 radioembolization using resin microspheres: a technical review. Ann Nucl Med 2011;25:455–461.
14 Kennedy A, Nag S, Salem R, Murthy R, McEwan AJ, Nutting C, Benson A 3rd, Espat J, Bilbao JI, Sharma RA, Thomas JP, Coldwell D: Recommendations for radioembolization of hepatic malignancies using yttrium-90 microsphere brachytherapy: a consensus panel report from the radioembolization brachytherapy oncology consortium. Int J Radiat Oncol Biol Phys 2007;68:13–23.
15 Wang SC, Bester L, Burnes JP, Clouston JE, Hugh TJ, Little AF, Padbury RT, Price D: Clinical care and technical recommendations for ^{90}yttrium microsphere treatment of liver cancer. J Med Imaging Radiat Oncol 2010;54:178–187.
16 Lau WY, Ho S, Leung TW, Chan M, Ho R, Johnson PJ, Li AK: Selective internal radiation therapy for nonresectable hepatocellular carcinoma with intraarterial infusion of ^{90}yttrium microspheres. Int J Radiat Oncol Biol Phys 1998;40:583–592.

17 Mazzaferro V, Sposito C, Bhoori S, Romito R, Chiesa C, Morosi C, Maccauro M, Marchiano A, Bongini M, Lanocita R, Civelli E, Bombardieri E, Camerini T, Spreafico C: Yttrium^{90} radioembolization for intermediate-advanced hepatocarcinoma: A phase II study. Hepatology 2012, E-pub ahead of print.
18 Salem R, Lewandowski RJ, Kulik L, Wang E, Riaz A, Ryu RK, Sato KT, Gupta R, Nikolaidis P, Miller FH, Yaghmai V, Ibrahim SM, Senthilnathan S, Baker T, Gates VL, Atassi B, Newman S, Memon K, Chen R, Vogelzang RL, Nemcek AA, Resnick SA, Chrisman HB, Carr J, Omary RA, Abecassis M, Benson AB 3rd, Mulcahy MF: Radioembolization results in longer time-to-progression and reduced toxicity compared with chemoembolization in patients with hepatocellular carcinoma. Gastroenterology 2011;140:497–507.
19 Hilgard P, Hamami M, Fouly AE, Scherag A, Muller S, Ertle J, Heusner T, Cicinnati VR, Paul A, Bockisch A, Gerken G, Antoch G: Radioembolization with yttrium-90 glass microspheres in hepatocellular carcinoma: European experience on safety and long-term survival. Hepatology 2010;52:1741–1749.
20 Tsai AL, Burke CT, Kennedy AS, Moore DT, Mauro MA, Dixon RD, Stavas JM, Bernard SA, Khandani AH, O'Neil BH: Use of yttrium-90 microspheres in patients with advanced hepatocellular carcinoma and portal vein thrombosis. J Vasc Interv Radiol 2010;21:1377–1384.
21 Salem R, Lewandowski RJ, Mulcahy MF, Riaz A, Ryu RK, Ibrahim S, Atassi B, Baker T, Gates V, Miller FH, Sato KT, Wang E, Gupta R, Benson AB, Newman SB, Omary RA, Abecassis M, Kulik L: Radioembolization for hepatocellular carcinoma using yttrium-90 microspheres: a comprehensive report of long-term outcomes. Gastroenterology 2010;138:52–64.
22 Riaz A, Lewandowski RJ, Kulik LM, Mulcahy MF, Sato KT, Ryu RK, Omary RA, Salem R: Complications following radioembolization with yttrium-90 microspheres: a comprehensive literature review. J Vasc Interv Radiol 2009;20:1121–1131.
23 Salem R, Lewandowski RJ, Atassi B, Gordon SC, Gates VL, Barakat O, Sergie Z, Wong CY, Thurston KG: Treatment of unresectable hepatocellular carcinoma with use of ^{90}Y microspheres (TheraSphere): safety, tumor response, and survival. J Vasc Interv Radiol 2005;16:1627–1639.
24 Kennedy AS, Coldwell D, Nutting C, Murthy R, Wertman DE Jr, Loehr SP, Overton C, Meranze S, Niedzwiecki J, Sailer S: Resin ^{90}Y-microsphere brachytherapy for unresectable colorectal liver metastases: modern USA experience. Int J Radiat Oncol Biol Phys 2006;65:412–425.
25 Sato K, Lewandowski RJ, Bui JT, Omary R, Hunter RD, Kulik L, Mulcahy M, Liu D, Chrisman H, Resnick S, Nemcek AA Jr, Vogelzang R, Salem R: Treatment of unresectable primary and metastatic liver cancer with yttrium-90 microspheres (TheraSphere): assessment of hepatic arterial embolization. Cardiovasc Intervent Radiol 2006;29:522–529.
26 Kennedy AS, McNeillie P, Dezarn WA, Nutting C, Sangro B, Wertman D, Garafalo M, Liu D, Coldwell D, Savin M, Jakobs T, Rose S, Warner R, Carter D, Sapareto S, Nag S, Gulec S, Calkins A, Gates VL, Salem R: Treatment parameters and outcome in 680 treatments of internal radiation with resin ^{90}Y-microspheres for unresectable hepatic tumors. Int J Radiat Oncol Biol Phys 2009;74:1494–1500.
27 Atassi B, Bangash AK, Lewandowski RJ, Ibrahim S, Kulik L, Mulcahy MF, Murthy R, Ryu RK, Sato KT, Miller FH, Omary RA, Salem R: Biliary sequelae following radioembolization with yttrium-90 microspheres. J Vasc Interv Radiol 2008;19:691–697.
28 Leung TW, Lau WY, Ho SK, Ward SC, Chow JH, Chan MS, Metreweli C, Johnson PJ, Li AK: Radiation pneumonitis after selective internal radiation treatment with intraarterial ^{90}yttrium-microspheres for inoperable hepatic tumors. Int J Radiat Oncol Biol Phys 1995;33:919–924.
29 Sangro B, Carpanese L, Cianni R, Golfieri R, Gasparini D, Ezziddin S, Paprottka PM, Fiore F, Van Buskirk M, Bilbao JI, Ettorre GM, Salvatori R, Giampalma E, Geatti O, Wilhelm K, Hoffmann RT, Izzo F, Inarrairaegui M, Maini CL, Urigo C, Cappelli A, Vit A, Ahmadzadehfar H, Jakobs TF, Lastoria S: Survival after yttrium-90 resin microsphere radioembolization of hepatocellular carcinoma across Barcelona Clinic Liver Cancer stages: a European evaluation. Hepatology 2011;54:868–878.
30 Lance C, McLennan G, Obuchowski N, Cheah G, Levitin A, Sands M, Spain J, Srinivas S, Shrikanthan S, Aucejo FN, Kim R, Menon KV: Comparative analysis of the safety and efficacy of transcatheter arterial chemoembolization and yttrium-90 radioembolization in patients with unresectable hepatocellular carcinoma. J Vasc Interv Radiol 2011;22:1697–1705.
31 Bruix J, Sherman M: Management of hepatocellular carcinoma: an update. Hepatology 2011;53:1020–1022.
32 Omata M, Lesmana LA, Tateishi R, Chen PJ, Lin SM, Yoshida H, Kudo M, Lee JM, Choi BI, Poon RT, Shiina S, Cheng AL, Jia JD, Obi S, Han KH, Jafri W, Chow P, Lim SG, Chawla YK, Budihusodo U, Gani RA, Lesmana CR, Putranto TA, Liaw YF, Sarin SK: Asian Pacific Association for the Study of the Liver consensus recommendations on hepatocellular carcinoma. Hepatol Int 2010;4:439–474.
33 Han KH, Kudo M, Ye SL, Choi JY, Poon RT, Seong J, Park JW, Ichida T, Chung JW, Chow P, Cheng AL: Asian consensus workshop report: expert consensus guideline for the management of intermediate and advanced hepatocellular carcinoma in Asia. Oncology 2011;81(suppl 1):158–164.
34 Han KH, Seong J, Kim JK, Ahn SH, Lee do Y, Chon CY: Pilot clinical trial of localized concurrent chemoradiation therapy for locally advanced hepatocellular carcinoma with portal vein thrombosis. Cancer 2008;113:995–1003.
35 Kulik LM, Carr BI, Mulcahy MF, Lewandowski RJ, Atassi B, Ryu RK, Sato KT, Benson A 3rd, Nemcek AA Jr, Gates VL, Abecassis M, Omary RA, Salem R: Safety and efficacy of ^{90}Y radiotherapy for hepatocellular carcinoma with and without portal vein thrombosis. Hepatology 2008;47:71–81.
36 Fox RA, Klemp PF, Egan G, Mina LL, Burton MA, Gray BN: Dose distribution following selective internal radiation therapy. Int J Radiat Oncol Biol Phys 1991;21:463–467.
37 Wigg A, Wallington M: Yttrium 90 therapy for hepatocellular carcinoma: is it any better than conventional external beam radiotherapy? Hepatology 2012;55:981–982.
38 Young JY, Rhee TK, Atassi B, Gates VL, Kulik L, Mulcahy MF, Larson AC, Ryu RK, Sato KT, Lewandowski RJ, Omary RA, Salem R: Radiation dose limits and liver toxicities resulting from multiple yttrium-90 radioembolization treatments for hepatocellular carcinoma. J Vasc Interv Radiol 2007;18:1375–1382.
39 Sangro B, Bilbao JI, Boan J, Martinez-Cuesta A, Benito A, Rodriguez J, Panizo A, Gil B, Inarrairaegui M, Herrero I, Quiroga J, Prieto J: Radioembolization using ^{90}Y-resin microspheres for patients with advanced hepatocellular carcinoma. Int J Radiat Oncol Biol Phys 2006;66:792–800.
40 Carr BI: Hepatic arterial ^{90}Yttrium glass microspheres (TheraSphere) for unresectable hepatocellular carcinoma: interim safety and survival data on 65 patients. Liver Transpl 2004;10:S107–S110.

Oncology

Oncology 2013;84(suppl 1):40–43
DOI: 10.1159/000345888

Published online: February 20, 2013

Transcatheter Arterial Chemoembolization Combined with Radiofrequency Ablation for the Treatment of Hepatocellular Carcinoma

Zhen-Wei Peng[a–c] Min-Shan Chen[a, b]

[a]State Key Laboratory of Oncology in Southern China, [b]Department of Hepatobiliary Surgery, Sun Yat-sen University Cancer Center, and [c]Department of Oncology, the First Affiliated Hospital, Sun Yat-sen University, Guangzhou, PR China

Key Words
Hepatocellular carcinoma · Radiofrequency ablation · Transcatheter arterial chemoembolization

Abstract
Radiofrequency ablation (RFA) has become an important treatment for hepatocellular carcinoma (HCC). Nowadays, RFA is generally recognized as an alternative treatment to partial hepatectomy for early HCC, especially for patients with impaired liver function and when liver transplantation is not indicated, although some authors consider that RFA can be used as a first-line treatment for early HCC. Transcatheter arterial chemoembolization (TACE) is most commonly classified as palliative rather than potentially curative; there is evidence that TACE prolongs survival in patients with well-compensated liver disease and intermediate-stage HCC. Alone, TACE and RFA have their limitations; in particular, neither can result in adequate control of medium or large HCC. Sequential application of TACE and RFA is, therefore, increasingly being used in the treatment of HCC in patients with well-compensated liver disease. In this study, we will introduce our experience of TACE combined with RFA in the treatment of HCC in a cancer center in China.

The incidence of hepatocellular carcinoma (HCC) has increased dramatically worldwide in the past decade, making it currently the sixth most common cancer in the world and the third most frequent cause of cancer death [1]. Although more patients with HCC are being diagnosed at an earlier stage by surveillance using ultrasonography and fetoprotein levels [2–4], most HCCs are diagnosed at intermediate or advanced stages, and only 30% of patients benefit from curative therapies such as resection, liver transplantation or percutaneous ablation [5, 6]. Until now, no standard therapy has been established for treatment of HCC [7–10]. Transcatheter arterial chemoembolization (TACE) and radiofrequency ablation (RFA) are minimally invasive options that may individually or in combination achieve the pertinent balance in successful tumor eradication and maximal preservation of liver function. TACE can slow tumor progression and improves survival by combining the effect of targeted chemotherapy with ischemic necrosis by arterial embolization [11, 12]. Although TACE is most commonly classified as palliative rather than potentially curative, there is evidence that TACE prolongs survival in patients with well-compensated liver disease and intermediate-stage HCC [13–16]. RFA has become an important treatment for HCC [17]. RFA has emerged as an accepted ther-

KARGER

Fax +41 61 306 12 34
E-Mail karger@karger.com
www.karger.com

0030–2414/13/0847–0040$38.00/0

Accessible online at:
www.karger.com/ocl

Min-Shan Chen, MD, PhD
Department of Hepatobiliary Surgery
Sun Yat-sen University Cancer Center
Guangzhou 510060 (PR China)
E-Mail Chminsh@mail.sysu.edu.cn

apy for early HCC because of its effectiveness and safety [18]. The optimum candidates for RFA are patients with HCC at an early stage (solitary tumor <5 cm in diameter or fewer than 3 nodules <3 cm in diameter). Nowadays, RFA is generally recognized as an alternative treatment to partial hepatectomy for early HCC, especially for patients with impaired liver function and when liver transplantation is not indicated, although some authors consider that RFA can be used as a first-line treatment for early HCC [10, 19, 20]. However, the likelihood of complete ablation using RFA declines rapidly as tumor diameter increases [21]. The complete response rate after RFA for HCC ≤2 cm is over 90%, but the local failure rate in individuals with HCC between 3.1 and 4 cm may be 24% with patients treated with RFA, and the likelihood of complete ablation rapidly declines beyond 4 cm [6]. Either TACE or RFA has its own limitations, in particular, neither can result in adequate control of medium or large HCC [6, 8–10, 13, 14]. Because blood flow promotes heat loss, and heat loss may reduce the effectiveness of RFA, a possible way to increase the ablation size of RFA thermal lesions would be to reduce or eliminate the heat loss that is mediated by tissue perfusion [21]. Blood flow to HCC lesions can be substantially reduced by the arterial embolization effect of TACE treatment. Moreover, TACE has a strong antitumor effect on HCC lesions. The synergy between TACE and RFA is well described [21, 22]. Occlusion of hepatic arterial flow by embolization reduces the cooling effect of hepatic blood flow on thermal coagulation. Furthermore, iodized oil and gelatin sponge particles used in TACE fill the peripheral portal vein around the tumor by going through multiple arterioportal communications [23, 24], thus reducing the portal venous flow. As a consequence, RFA can enable the creation of larger thermal lesions by RFA. The effect of chemotherapeutic anticancer agents on cancer cells enhances the effect of hyperthermia [25]. TACE, being a regional treatment, can target undetected satellite lesions outside of the zone of RFA-induced necrosis. Moreover, disruption of intratumoral septa, which usually happens after TACE, facilitates heat distribution within the tumor, and intratumoral septa and fibrosis are considered to hamper heat diffusion within the tumor [26]. Sequential application of TACE and RFA is, therefore, increasingly being used in the treatment of HCC in patients with well-compensated liver disease.

Recently, some studies have compared the efficacy of combined TACE and RFA with RFA alone for the treatment of HCC. A recently published randomized controlled trial by Shibata et al. [27] demonstrated a survival equality for combined TACE and RFA (n = 46) compared with RFA alone (n = 43) in patients with Child's A or B cirrhosis and resectable HCC with ≤3 nodules smaller than 3 cm. In this study, after treatment, the 1-, 2-, 3- and 4-year rates of local tumor progression, overall survival, local progression-free survival and recurrence-free survival were as follows: local tumor progression rates were 14.4, 17.6, 17.6 and 17.6%, respectively, in the combined treatment group and 11.4, 14.4, 14.4 and 14.4%, respectively, in the RFA group ($p = 0.797$). Overall survival rates were 100, 100, 84.8 and 72.7%, respectively, in the combined treatment group and 100, 88.8, 84.5 and 74.0%, respectively, in the RFA group ($p = 0.515$). Local progression-free survival rates were 84.6, 81.1, 69.7 and 55.8%, respectively, in the combined treatment group and 88.4, 74.1, 74.1 and 61.7%, respectively, in the RFA group ($p = 0.934$). Event-free survival rates were 71.3, 59.9, 48.8 and 36.6%, respectively, in the combined treatment group and 74.3, 52.4, 29.7 and 29.7%, respectively, in the RFA group ($p = 0.365$). In light of this study, the authors considered that combined RFA plus TACE and RFA alone have equivalent effectiveness for the treatment of small (≤3 cm) HCCs, and they thought the combination treatment may not be necessary. In the study, both treatment groups had low rates of major complications (2.2–2.3%) and it was stated that treatment of HCC by combined TACE and RFA was safe. Morimoto et al. [28] reported the midterm outcomes of a randomized controlled trial comparing the efficacy of TACE combined with RFA with RFA alone for the treatment of intermediate-sized HCC. In the study, the authors randomly assigned 37 patients with solitary HCCs (diameter 3.1–5.0 cm in the greatest dimension) to 2 groups: the TACE combined with RFA (TACE-RFA) group, and the RFA group. The results showed that technical success was achieved after 1.4 ± 0.5 RFA sessions in the RFA group and after 1.1 ± 0.2 RFA sessions in the TACE-RFA group ($p < 0.01$). The mean diameters of the longer and shorter axes of the RFA-induced ablated areas were 50 ± 8.0 and 41 ± 7.1 mm, respectively, in the RFA group and 58 ± 13.2 and 50 ± 11.3 mm, respectively, in the TACE-RFA group; the mean diameters of the shorter axes were significantly different ($p = 0.012$). The rates of local tumor progression at the end of the third year in the RFA and TACE-RFA groups were 39 and 6%, respectively ($p = 0.012$). The 3-year survival rates of the patients in the RFA and TACE-RFA groups were 80 and 93%, respectively ($p = 0.369$). The authors reported that TACE prior to RFA expanded the short axis of the ablated area and resulted in a more spherical ablated area. They postulated that a spherical ablated area was more effective than a nonspherical ablated area in ensuring local tumor control because a spherical ablated area was more likely to completely cover the target tumor. TACE-RFA was also a safe treatment in this study. The result showed that there were no severe side effects during the procedures in the study; however, 6 patients (5 patients of the RFA group and 1 patient of the TACE-RFA group) experienced grade 1–2 pain lasting several hours. Major complications were not observed in the patients of the 2 groups. Minor complications, including asymptomatic right pleural effusion, were noted within 3 days of the procedures in 2 patients of the RFA group and 1 patient of the TACE-RFA group (RFA group vs. TACE-RFA group, $p = 0.515$). Therefore, the role of TACE combined with RFA in the treatment of HCC needs further study.

Recently, some authors have used meta-analysis to verify the role of TACE combined with RFA in the treatment of HCC. In the work of Yan et al. [29], 19 studies (including 4 randomized control trials) were included into the meta-analysis. Meta-analyses showed that the combination of RFA and TACE was associated with higher survival rates (1-year OR = 2.14, 95% CI 1.57–2.91, $p = 0.001$; 3-year OR = 1.98, 95% CI 1.28–3.07, $p = 0.001$; 5-year OR = 2.70, 95% CI 1.42–5.14, $p = 0.003$). They postulate that the combination of TACE with RFA can improve the overall survival rate and provide better prognosis for patients with HCC, but more randomized controlled trials using large sample size are needed to provide sufficient evidence. In another meta-analysis study, Wang et al. [30] reported that there was no survival benefit from TACE combined with RFA in treating small HCC (≤3 cm) patients as compared with that of RFA alone. The advantages of TACE-RFA may be as follows: TACE can block the hepatic arterial flow and contribute to the decrease in heat-sink effects and the increase in the necrotic area induced by RFA, and the effect of anticancer agents on cancer cells may be enhanced by the hyperthermia. However, these advantages do not seem to have any indication according to Wang et al's [29] meta-analysis for small HCC. The reason for this may be that RFA has already achieved complete necrosis in >90% in treating small HCC nodules [31], suggesting that adding TACE to RFA seems to be redundant in producing an assessed outcome. Schwartz and Weintraub [32] considered that the clearest role for the combination of TACE and RFA is to increase the likelihood of complete destruction of HCC nodules that are in the range of 3–5 cm. They also say that patients selected for combined TACE and RFA should have well-compensated cirrhosis, and the rationale for using combined therapy is strongest for patients with uninodular HCC.

We agree with that idea. Recently, a randomized controlled trial published by us demonstrated that the survival benefit for combined TACE and RFA ($n = 94$) was comparable with RFA alone ($n = 95$) in patients with Child's A or B cirrhosis and resectable HCC with ≤3 nodules smaller than 7 cm [33]. In our study, after treatment, the 1-, 3- and 4-year overall survival rates for the TACE-RFA group and the RFA group were 92.6, 66.6 and 61.8%, and 85.3, 59 and 45.0%, respectively. The corresponding recurrence-free survival rates were 79.4, 60.6 and 54.8%, and 66.7, 44.2 and 38.9%, respectively. Patients in the TACE-RFA group had better overall survival and recurrence-free survival than the RFA group ($p = 0.002$ and 0.009, respectively). After multivariate analysis, treatment allocation, tumor size and tumor number were significant prognostic factors for overall survival, while treatment allocation and tumor number were significant prognostic factors for recurrence-free survival. There were no treatment-related deaths in this study. In light of this study, the role of combined TACE and RFA warrants careful consideration. The study provides evidence that altering the tumor microenvironment and supporting vasculature may help improve the efficacy of locoregional therapy in HCC. We therefore think that, in the future, the standard of care for HCC treatable with RFA should shift toward the combination treatment. We know that RFA has already begun to challenge the status of resection as the optimum treatment for HCC ≤2 cm; combined RFA and TACE will certainly broaden this challenge. In the future, further logical studies will be to investigate the potential benefit offered by complementary treatment modalities, such as targeted agents in combination with TACE-RFA [11, 12].

Disclosure Statement

This work is supported by the grant from the State Key Project on Infectious Diseases of China (Grant No. 2012ZX10002-016), and the 5010 Foundation of Sun Yat-sen University (Grant No. 2007043).

References

1 Jemal A, Bray F, Center MM, Ferlay J, Ward E, Forman D: Global cancer statistics. CA Cancer J Clin 2011;61:69–90.

2 Bruix J, Llovet JM: HCC surveillance: who is the target population? Hepatology 2003;37: 507–509.

3 Kudo M: Japan's Successful Model of Nationwide Hepatocellular Carcinoma Surveillance Highlighting the Urgent Need for Global Surveillance. Liver Cancer, in press.

4 Kim DY, Han KH: Epidemiology and surveillance of hepatocellular carcinoma. Liver Cancer 2012;1:2–14.

5 Bruix J, Llovet JM: Prognostic prediction and treatment strategy in hepatocellular carcinoma. Hepatology 2002;35:519–24.

6 Llovet JM, Burroughs A, Bruix J: Hepatocellular carcinoma. Lancet 2003;362:1907–1917.

7 Lin SM, Lin CJ, Lin CC, Hsu CW, Chen YC: Radiofrequency ablation improves prognosis compared with ethanol injection for hepatocellular carcinoma ≤ 4 cm. Gastroenterology 2004;127:1714–1723.

8 Llovet JM, Bruix J: Systematic review of randomized trials for unresectable hepatocellular carcinoma: chemoembolization improves survival. Hepatology 2003;37:429–442.

9 Takayasu K, Arii S, Ikai I, Omata M, Okita K, Ichida T, et al: Prospective cohort study of transarterial chemoembolization for unresectable hepatocellular carcinoma in 8,510 patients. Gastroenterology 2006;131:461–469.

10 Chen MS, Li JQ, Zheng Y, Guo RP, Liang HH, Zhang YQ, et al: A prospective randomized trial comparing percutaneous local ablative therapy and partial hepatectomy for small hepatocellular carcinoma. Ann Surg 2006; 243:321–328.

11 Hsu C, Liang PC, Morita S, Hu FC, Cheng AL: Perspectives on the design of clinical trials combining transarterial chemoembolization and molecular targeted therapy. Liver Cancer, in press.

12 Liapi E, Geschwind JF: Combination of local transcatheter arterial chemoembolization and systemic anti-angiogenic therapy for unresectable hepatocellular carcinoma. Liver Cancer, in press.

13 Llovet JM, Real MI, Montana X, Planas R, Coll S, Aponte J, et al: Arterial embolisation or chemoembolisation versus symptomatic treatment in patients with unresectable hepatocellular carcinoma: a randomised controlled trial. Lancet 2002;359:1734–1739.

14 Lo CM, Ngan H, Tso WK, Liu CL, Lam CM, Poon RT, et al: Randomized controlled trial of transarterial lipiodol chemoembolization for unresectable hepatocellular carcinoma. Hepatology 2002;35:1164–1171.

15 Lencioni R: Chemoembolization in patients with hepatocellular carcinoma. Liver Cancer 2012;1:41–50.

16 Lin S, Hoffmann K, Schemmer P: Treatment of hepatocellular carcinoma: a systematic review. Liver Cancer, in press.

17 Salvatore V, Bolondi L: Clinical impact of ultrasound-related techniques in the diagnosis of focal liver lesions. Liver Cancer, in press.

18 Chen MS, Zhang YJ, Li JQ: The role of radiofrequency ablation in treating small hepatocellular carcinoma. Chin J Cancer 2007;26: 449–152.

19 Livraghi T, Meloni F, Di Stasi M, Rolle E, Solbiati L, Tinelli C, et al: Sustained complete response and complications rates after radiofrequency ablation of very early hepatocellular carcinoma in cirrhosis: is resection still the treatment of choice? Hepatology 2008;47:82–89.

20 Rossi S, Ravetta V, Rosa L, Ghittoni G, Viera FT, Garbagnati F, et al: Repeated radiofrequency ablation for management of patients with cirrhosis with small hepatocellular carcinomas: a long-term cohort study. Hepatology 2011;53:136–147.

21 Rossi S, Garbagnati F, Lencioni R, Allgaier HP, Marchiano A, Fornari F, et al: Percutaneous radio-frequency thermal ablation of nonresectable hepatocellular carcinoma after occlusion of tumor blood supply. Radiology 2000;217:119–126.

22 Ganbold U, Kim YH, Cho SB, Kim GM, Chung HH: Combined TACE and RFA treatment of HCC lesion in contact with blood vessels: local recurrence due to heat sink effect. Liver Cancer 2012;1:117.

23 Seki T, Wakabayashi M, Nakagawa T, Itho T, Shiro T, Kunieda K, et al: Ultrasonically guided percutaneous microwave coagulation therapy for small hepatocellular carcinoma. Cancer 1994;74:817–825.

24 Seki T, Tamai T, Nakagawa T, Imamura M, Nishimura A, Yamashiki N, et al: Combination therapy with transcatheter arterial chemoembolization and percutaneous microwave coagulation therapy for hepatocellular carcinoma. Cancer 2000;89:1245–1251.

25 Higuchi T, Kikuchi M, Okazaki M: Hepatocellular carcinoma after transcatheter hepatic arterial embolization: a histopathologic study of 84 resected cases. Cancer 1994;73: 2259–2267.

26 Nakashima Y, Nakashima O, Hsia CC, Kojiro M, Tabor E: Vascularization of small hepatocellular carcinomas: correlation with differentiation. Liver 1999;19:12–18.

27 Shibata T, Isoda H, Hirokawa Y, Arizono S, Shimada K, Togashi K: Small hepatocellular carcinoma: is radiofrequency ablation combined with transcatheter arterial chemoembolization more effective than radiofrequency ablation alone for treatment? Radiology 2009;252:905–913.

28 Morimoto M, Numata K, Kondou M, Nozaki A, Morita S, Tanaka K: Midterm outcomes in patients with intermediate-sized hepatocellular carcinoma: a randomized controlled trial for determining the efficacy of radiofrequency ablation combined with transcatheter arterial chemoembolization. Cancer 2010;116:5452–5460.

29 Yan S, Xu D, Sun B: Combination of radiofrequency ablation with transarterial chemoembolization for hepatocellular carcinoma: a meta-analysis. Dig Dis Sci 2012;57: 3026–3031.

30 Wang W, Shi J, Xie WF: Transarterial chemoembolization in combination with percutaneous ablation therapy in unresectable hepatocellular carcinoma: a meta-analysis. Liver Int 2010;30:741–749.

31 Shibata T, Maetani Y, Isoda H, Hiraoka M: Radiofrequency ablation for small hepatocellular carcinoma: prospective comparison of internally cooled electrode and expandable electrode. Radiology 2006;238:346–353.

32 Schwartz M, Weintraub J: Combined transarterial chemoembolization and radiofrequency ablation for hepatocellular carcinoma. Nat Clin Pract Oncol 2008;5:630–631.

33 Peng ZW, Zhang YJ, Chen MS, Xu L, Liang HH, Lin XJ, et al: Radiofrequency ablation with or without transcatheter arterial chemoembolization in the treatment of hepatocellular carcinoma: a prospective randomized trial. J Clin Oncol, in press.

Oncology

Oncology 2013;84(suppl 1):44–50
DOI: 10.1159/000345889

Published online: February 20, 2013

Ultrasonography Fusion Imaging System Increases the Chance of Radiofrequency Ablation for Hepatocellular Carcinoma with Poor Conspicuity on Conventional Ultrasonography

Yuki Makino[a] Yasuharu Imai[a] Hideko Ohama[a] Takumi Igura[a] Sachiyo Kogita[a] Yoshiyuki Sawai[a] Kazuto Fukuda[a] Manabu Takamura[b] Hiroshi Ohashi[c] Takamichi Murakami[d]

Departments of [a]Gastroenterology, [b]Radiology and [c]Pathology, Ikeda Municipal Hospital, Ikeda, and [d]Department of Radiology, Kinki University School of Medicine, Osakasayama, Japan

Key Words

Ultrasonography fusion imaging · Multimodality fusion imaging · Volume Navigation System · Hepatocellular carcinoma · Radiofrequency ablation

Abstract

Objectives: To investigate the usefulness of the ultrasonography (US) fusion imaging system for radiofrequency ablation (RFA) for hepatocellular carcinoma (HCC). ***Methods:*** Since the US fusion imaging system became available in 2010, we have conducted RFA with this system in all cases. The characteristics of 75 patients with 120 HCCs and 89 patients with 123 HCCs who underwent RFA before the introduction of this system (period A) and after it (period B), respectively, were retrospectively compared. ***Results:*** Significant difference in the characteristics of the patients and HCCs between the two periods was found only in the proportion of HCCs with poor conspicuity on grayscale US treated with RFA (1.7%, 2/120 for period A vs. 15.4%, 19/123 for period B, $p < 0.01$). Among the 19 HCCs with poor conspicuity on grayscale US for period B, 5 and 9 HCCs were identified on grayscale US and contrast-enhanced US, respectively, by the use of the US fusion imaging system, whereas the 5 remaining undetectable HCCs were treated by using the system in conjunction with reference images displayed side-by-side with grayscale US. ***Conclusion:*** Since the introduction of the US fusion imaging system, it has become possible to perform RFA for HCCs with poor conspicuity on grayscale US.

Introduction

Hepatocellular carcinoma (HCC), usually developing from chronic liver diseases such as hepatitis B- and C-related cirrhosis, is one of the most common cancer types worldwide [1, 2]. The treatments for HCC are usually determined on the basis of staging and hepatic functional reserve. Loco-regional treatments such as radiofrequency ablation (RFA) and percutaneous ethanol injection therapy are indicated, in principal, for HCCs up to 3 nodules and 3 cm in diameter [3–5]. Although percutaneous ethanol injection therapy is preferred in certain situations where it is difficult to perform RFA, such as for tumors surrounded by large vessels [6], RFA is now established as the first-choice loco-regional treatment, since RFA is considered superior to percutaneous ethanol injection therapy in terms of the local tumor progression and overall survival rates [7].

KARGER

Fax +41 61 306 12 34
E-Mail karger@karger.com
www.karger.com

0030–2414/13/0847–0044$38.00/0

Accessible online at:
www.karger.com/ocl

Yasuharu Imai, MD, PhD
Department of Gastroenterology,
Ikeda Municipal Hospital
3-1-18, Johnan, Ikeda, Osaka 563-8510 (Japan)
E-Mail yasuimai@hosp.ikeda.osaka.jp

Since second-generation contrast medium for ultrasonography (US) including Sonazoid (Daiichi-sankyo, Tokyo, Japan) and gadolinium ethoxybenzyl diethylenetriamine pentaacetic acid (Gd-EOB-DTPA; Primovist, Bayer Healthcare, Osaka, Japan), a liver-specific magnetic resonance (MR) contrast agent, became available, imaging diagnosis of HCC has dramatically advanced [8–14]. As a result, the diagnosis of HCC has come to be made at an earlier stage. If HCCs are diagnosed at an early stage, RFA is often one of the treatment options. However, since early HCCs are sometimes difficult to detect on conventional US, we are obliged to give up conducting RFA.

The US fusion imaging system, which has recently been introduced for the assistance of loco-regional treatment for HCC, can show real-time US images and any cross-sectional multiplanar reconstruction images of CT or MRI synchronously, side-by-side. The US fusion imaging system has been reported to be useful for the detection of HCC with poor conspicuity on conventional US [15–17]. Therefore, even if a targeted tumor is not conspicuous on conventional US, percutaneous loco-regional treatment can be applied by using the US fusion imaging system.

The purpose of this study was to retrospectively compare the characteristics of the patients and tumors which underwent RFA, before and after the introduction of the US fusion imaging system, in order to verify the improvement in the practice of RFA for HCC yielded by this system.

Materials and Methods

Patients and HCCs

This retrospective study was approved by our institutional review board and informed consent for this study was waived. Consecutive patients with HCC who underwent RFA from September 2009 to January 2011 were enrolled in this study.

The diagnosis of hypervascular HCC was established on the basis of the typical imaging features on dynamic CT, CT angiography or Gd-EOB-DTPA-enhanced MRI [10]. Tumor biopsy was conducted for the nodules which were more than 10 mm in diameter and showed hypointensity on the hepatobiliary phase of Gd-EOB-DTPA-enhanced MRI without early enhancement, on at least two imaging modalities of contrast-enhanced US (CEUS), dynamic CT and Gd-EOB-DTPA-enhanced MRI [9, 18]. Pathological diagnosis of HCC was made according to the histological criteria of the International Consensus Group for Hepatocellular Carcinoma [18].

Needle Core Biopsy and RFA Procedures

Needle core biopsy and RFA were performed by one of 3 hepatologists with more than 10 years of experience. All needle core biopsy and RFA procedures were undertaken percutaneously under the US guidance of Aplio XG (Toshiba, Tokyo, Japan) from September 2009 to April 2010 (period A) and LOGIQ E9 (GE Healthcare Japan, Tokyo, Japan) equipped with the US fusion imaging system (Volume Navigation System, GE Healthcare Japan) from May 2010 to January 2011 (period B). At needle core biopsy, at least 2 samples were taken from each tumor using a 21-gauge needle (Majima needle, Top, Tokyo, Japan) to ensure accurate pathological diagnosis as described previously [19]. We used a 17-gauge cool-tip single electrode with a 2- or 3-cm exposed tip (Cool-tip RF Ablation System, Covidien, Colo., USA). We used artificial ascites or pleural effusion for tumors located on the liver surface, in the hepatic dome or adjacent to the gastrointestinal tract.

After applying a local anesthesia, an electrode was inserted into the tumor and ablation was initiated. Power output was first set at 20 or 30 W, respectively, for the 2- or 3-cm active tip of the electrode, and increased by 10 W/min until roll-off. Ablation was maintained at the energy level just before the first roll-off, until the fifth roll-off occurred, or until 12 min had elapsed since the start of ablation. We also ablated the needle track during the withdrawal of the electrode in order to prevent hemorrhage and tumor dissemination. With the aim of achieving the complete necrosis of the tumor, additional ablation was conducted when necessary.

Follow-Up after RFA

Dynamic CT was performed within 7 days after RFA and the treatment effect was evaluated comparing pre-RFA CT or MRI and post-RFA CT. If tumor stain was not recognized around the coagulated area in the arterial phase and the coagulated area was considered to circumferentially extend beyond the pre-RFA tumor boundary in the portal and equilibrium phases, it was judged to be completely ablated. If an obvious residual tumor was observed, additional treatment sessions were carried out until complete ablation was achieved. After complete ablation, a follow-up US, dynamic CT or Gd-EOB-DTPA-enhanced MRI and blood tests including tumor markers were performed every 3 months.

US Fusion Imaging System

From May 2010 to January 2011 (period B), we used Volume Navigation System installed in LOGIQ E9 for the assistance of RFA for all cases as described previously [20]. As reference images for Volume Navigation System, the imaging modality on which the tumor and landmarks for the positional registration were most clearly depicted was chosen.

After the volume data of CT or MR images for reference was imported as digital imaging and communication in medicine format, the cross-section of US images approximately parallel to the reference was registered. Then, one characteristic corresponding landmark between US images and reference was marked, respectively, and the position was aligned. In order to improve the registration accuracy, particularly around the tumor, the positional registration was repeatedly carried out as close to the tumor as possible. After the positional registration, multiplanar reconstruction images of CT or MRI were synchronously displayed side-by-side with the real-time US images.

Image Acquisition

Dynamic CT and CT Angiography

Dynamic CT and CT angiography were performed with either the 8-channel multidetector row helical CT (MDCT; LightSpeed Ultra, GE healthcare Japan) from September 2009 to September

2010, or the 64-channel MDCT (Discovery CT 750HD, GE healthcare Japan) from October 2010 to January 2011, with a slice thickness of 0.675 or 1.25 mm. In the dynamic CT the bolus tracking method was used for scanning, using 2.0 ml/kg of nonionic contrast material with a concentration of 300 gI/ml administered intravenously for 30 s with an automatic power injector. Images were obtained at approximately 35–45, 65–80 and 190–205 s, after starting the injection of the contrast agents for the arterial, portal and equilibrium phases, respectively [9].

For CT angiography, selective catheterization was conducted with two catheters inserted by the Seldinger technique from either the right or left femoral artery. One was placed in the superior mesenteric artery for CT during arterioportography and the other in the common hepatic artery for CT during hepatic arteriography. The former images were scanned 30–33 s after administration of 66–80 ml of 150–160 mgI/ml nonionic contrast agents at a rate of 2.0 ml/s. The latter images were scanned 5–8 s after injection of 20–33 ml of 150–160 mgI/ml nonionic contrast agents at a speed of 1.0 ml/s [19].

Gd-EOB-DTPA-Enhanced MRI

Gd-EOB-DTPA-enhanced MR imaging was performed using a 1.5-T system (Signa Excite HD 1.5T, GE Healthcare Japan) with a slice thickness of 3 or 5 mm. For the contrast enhancement, 25 μmol/kg body weight (0.1 ml/kg) of Gd-EOB-DTPA (Primovist, Bayer-Schering Pharma AG, Berlin, Germany) was administered intravenously at a rate of 2.0 ml/s. At first, an unenhanced MRI was obtained using a T1-weighted gradient echo sequence (dual echoes; in-phase and out-of-phase). Then, unenhanced, arterial, portal, late and hepatobiliary phase images were acquired just before, 25, 70, 180 s and 20 min, respectively, after injection of the contrast agent [9, 10].

Grayscale US and CEUS

The ultrasound systems used for the imaging of both grayscale US and CEUS were Aplio XG with a 3.5 MHz curved array convex probe or a 3.5 MHz microconvex probe from September 2009 to April 2010 (period A) or LOGIQE9 equipped with Volume Navigation System with a 3.5-MHz curved array convex probe or a 1- to 6-MHz microconvex probe from May 2010 to January 2011 (period B).

Before RFA, an attempt was made to detect all HCCs on grayscale US at first. The operator sought the tumor, carefully referencing the intrahepatic structures such as blood vessels, cysts or scars from previous treatments.

If the HCC could not be detected on grayscale US, CEUS using Sonazoid was conducted next, with or without the US fusion imaging (periods A and B, respectively), focusing on the site where the target tumor was likely to be depicted. Images of the vascular phase were acquired over a 120-second period with a low mechanical index of less than 0.3 after injection of 0.0075 ml/kg of Sonazoid. Images of the postvascular phase were obtained more than 10 min after administration of the contrast agent. If a hypoechoic area suggesting the tumor was observed in the postvascular phase, the same dose of Sonazoid was reinjected and the vascularity was evaluated [11].

Since LOGIQE9 was introduced in May 2010 (period B), grayscale US was carried out in order to identify a target tumor without Volume Navigation System at first. Subsequently, all procedures described above were conducted with Volume Navigation System in all cases. Detection of the HCCs by grayscale US and CEUS was assessed by the consensus of two hepatologists with more than 10 years of experience in abdominal ultrasonography.

Statistical Analysis

The characteristics of HCCs which underwent RFA before and after the introduction of Volume Navigation System were compared. The χ^2 statistic was used for the categorical data analysis and the Mann-Whitney U test was used for comparing the distribution of continuous variables. The data were analyzed using SPSS version 17.0 software (SPSS, Chicago, Ill., USA) and p value <0.05 was considered statistically significant.

Results

A total of 164 patients with 243 HCCs underwent RFA between September 2009 and January 2011. Regarding major complications, intercostal artery hemorrhage was observed in 2 cases (1.2%). All of the treated tumors were considered to be completely ablated on follow-up dynamic CT at the end, after one or more treatment sessions.

Patient and Tumor Characteristics

Between September 2009 and April 2010 (period A), 75 patients with 120 HCCs underwent RFA without the US fusion imaging system. Eighty-nine patients with 123 HCCs were treated with RFA with Volume Navigation System between May 2010 and January 2011 (period B). Clinical characteristics of the subjects are listed in table 1. There was no significant difference in the number of HCCs treated with RFA per case, the proportion of cases using artificial ascites or pleural effusion, and number of treatment sessions between periods A and B. However, the proportion of tumors with poor conspicuity on grayscale US significantly increased from 1.7 (2/120) to 15.4% (19/123) after the introduction of Volume Navigation System.

RFA for HCCs with Poor Conspicuity on Grayscale US Using the US Fusion Imaging System

If a tumor was difficult to visualize on grayscale US, CEUS was subsequently conducted. Before the introduction of Volume Navigation System (period A), images of vascular phase and postvascular phase were obtained by focusing on the site where the HCC was likely to be visualized, estimated from axial images of CT or MRI. However, only 2 HCCs could be detected on CEUS and treated with RFA in this way. If a tumor could not be detected either on grayscale US or CEUS, we were obliged to give up RFA.

Table 1. Characteristics of the patients and HCCs that underwent RFA with and without the US fusion imaging system

Variables	Without US fusion imaging system (period A)	With US fusion imaging system (period B)	p value
Patients, n	75	89	n.a.
HCCs, n	120	123	n.a.
HCCs treated with RFA per case, n	1.39 ± 0.76	1.37 ± 0.66	n.s.[a]
Mean tumor diameter, mm	15.8 ± 6.7	14.1 ± 6.2	n.s.[a]
HCCs using artificial ascites or pleural effusion, n	77 (64.2%)	90 (73.2%)	n.s.[b]
HCCs with poor conspicuity on grayscale US, n	2 (1.7%)	19 (15.4%)	<0.01[b]
Treatment sessions, n	1.07 ± 0.26	1.11 ± 0.33	n.s.[a]

[a] Mann-Whitney U test. [b] χ^2 statistic.

Meanwhile, 19 HCCs with poor conspicuity on grayscale US could be treated with RFA after the introduction of Volume Navigation System (period B). Among the 19 HCCs, 5 and 9 HCCs could be identified on grayscale US and CEUS, respectively, using Volume Navigation System. Nevertheless, the remaining 5 HCCs could not be detected either on grayscale US or CEUS with this system. However, we could carry out RFA on them with the assistance of Volume Navigation System, referencing the intrahepatic structures and hepatic contours on side-by-side images and aiming at the sites where tumors were expected to be located, or using the global positioning system (GPS) function, as described later.

Among the HCCs that underwent RFA with Volume Navigation System (period B), the diameter of tumors detectable on grayscale US (14.3 ± 6.7 mm, n = 104) was not different from that of HCCs with poor conspicuity on it (15.1 ± 6.8 mm, n = 19). In addition, the number of treatment sessions is also not different between the detectable HCCs and those with poor conspicuity. Accordingly, although the diameter of the HCCs with poor conspicuity on grayscale US was the same as that of detectable HCCs, they could be treated with RFA successfully in a single session in most cases, by virtue of Volume Navigation System.

Discussion

In recent years, the US fusion imaging system for the guidance of RFA has become available [8, 17, 20, 21]. In the US fusion imaging system, any cross-sectional multiplanar reconstruction images of the volume data of CT or MRI are synchronously displayed side-by-side with the real-time US images, in accordance with the movement of the probe [15–17, 20]. In this report, we have clearly shown that the number of HCCs with poor conspicuity on grayscale US and treated with RFA successfully has significantly increased since the introduction of the US fusion imaging system.

Gd-EOB-DTPA-enhanced MRI has been reported to have significantly higher sensitivity and diagnostic accuracy for detection of hypervascular HCC compared with multiphasic MDCT, particularly for small HCC, because of the additional effect of hepatobiliary phase images to dynamic images [10, 22]. It is also reported that Gd-EOB-DTPA-enhanced MRI is the most useful imaging technique for the detection of early HCC [9, 23, 24]. Accordingly, the opportunity to find small HCCs has increased since Gd-EOB-DTPA-enhanced MRI became available.

As to the local control after RFA, small HCCs are considered to be a good candidate for RFA, because local tumor progression after RFA is related to the tumor diameter [25]. However, RFA is usually conducted under US guidance, so it seems difficult to perform RFA in cases where tumor is hardly detectable on conventional US. Since the detection of HCC by US is considered to be related to the tumor size, in addition to the heterogeneous parenchymal echotexture of cirrhotic liver, it might not be easy to identify small HCCs on conventional US and perform RFA, even if they are diagnosed at an early stage by other imaging modalities such as Gd-EOB-DTPA-enhanced MRI [26–28].

CEUS with Sonazoid is reported to be useful for the diagnosis and treatment of HCC [8, 11, 29, 30]. Sonazoid provides a fine vascular image of hepatic tumors in vascular phase, and is very sensitive in detecting an early stain of HCC. Perfusion defect of HCC obtained in the postvascular phase is also useful for the detection of HCC. However, on the post-vascular phase of CEUS with

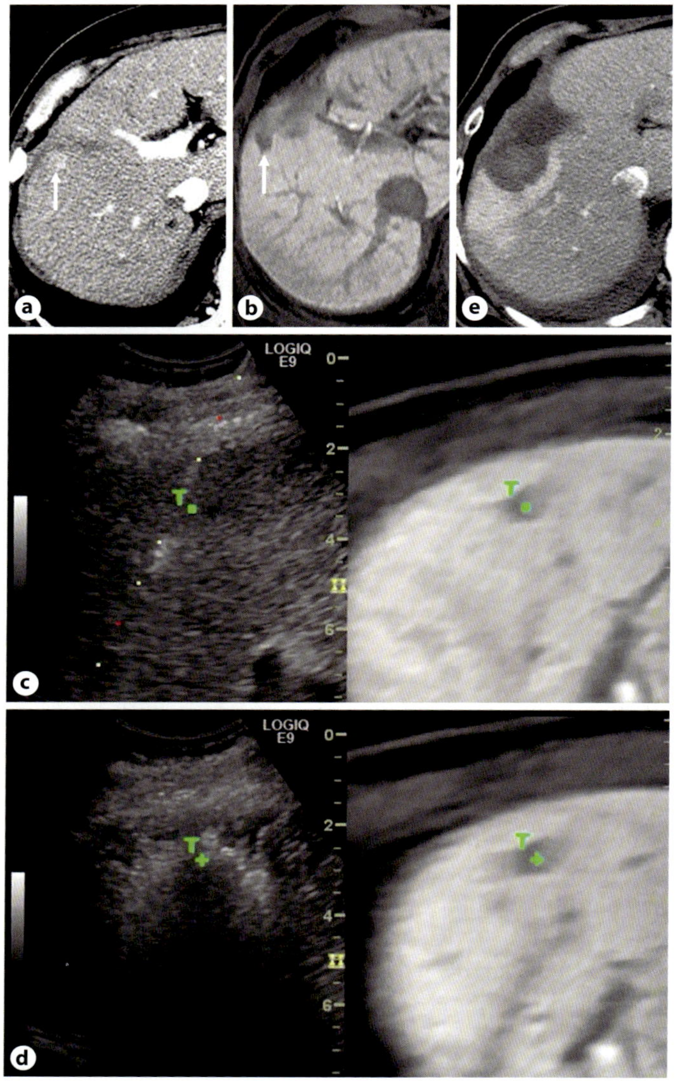

Fig. 1. RFA for HCC undetectable on US with guidance from the US fusion imaging system in a 63-year-old man. **a** Arterial phase of dynamic CT. **b** Hepatobiliary phase of Gd-EOB-DTPA-enhanced MRI. **c** Fusion images of grayscale US (left side) and hepatobiliary phase of Gd-EOB-DTPA-enhanced MRI (right side) using Volume Navigation System. **d** Fusion images of grayscale US just after RFA (left side) and hepatobiliary phase of Gd-EOB-DTPA-enhanced MRI (right side) using Volume Navigation System. **e** Portal phase of dynamic CT after RFA. HCC 13 mm in diameter in segment VIII could be depicted as a hypervascular and hypointense nodule on dynamic CT (**a**) and hepatobiliary phase of Gd-EOB-DTPA-enhanced MRI (**b**), respectively (arrows). However, it could not be depicted either on grayscale US or contrast-enhanced US, even with the assistance of Volume Navigation System. Thereupon, with the GPS function, the location of the targeted tumor on grayscale US was estimated in reference to the GPS marker, which indicated the tumor. RFA was then conducted by aiming at the site. Just after RFA, the tumor was considered to be fully encompassed within the high echoic bubbles of the ablation zone using the GPS function, suggesting complete ablation. Dynamic CT after RFA also indicated complete ablation, after a single treatment session.

Sonazoid, some well-differentiated HCCs do not show hypoechoic appearance and HCCs distant from the body surface are difficult to detect because of the signal attenuation, which is considered to be the limitation of CEUS with Sonazoid [31, 32].

The noteworthy usefulness of the US fusion imaging system is the detectability of HCCs with poor conspicuity on grayscale US. Although RFA is carried out under US guidance of intercostal scanning in most cases, it is often difficult to guess how a tumor is observed from the intercostal view from the axial images of CT or MRI. Hence, it does not seem easy to identify the locus of the targeted tumor unless it is well defined on grayscale US. However, with the US fusion imaging system, even if the targeted tumor is not conspicuous or surrounded by confusing cirrhosis-related nodules, it can be identified with confidence by comparing it with intrahepatic structures around the tumor on reference images. Kunishi et al. [17] and Lee et al. [21] also reported that the detection rate of HCC on grayscale US had increased by virtue of Volume Navigation System, which is consistent with our results. Moreover, some hypervascular HCCs not detected on conventional US have been reported to become detectable on the post-vascular phase of CEUS with Sonazoid [11]. Actually, 9 out of 19 tumors which underwent RFA with poor conspicuity on grayscale US could be identified combining CEUS and the US fusion imaging system in this study (period B), whereas only 2 HCCs with poor conspicuity on grayscale US could be detected on CEUS and treated with RFA before the introduction of the system (period A). Another 5 of the 19 HCCs of period B could be detected on grayscale US, using Volume Navigation System.

Finally, 5 out of 19 HCCs with poor conspicuity on grayscale US of period B could not be detected in spite of the use of the US fusion imaging system. This is considered to be partly because of the limitation of CEUS, as described above. However, even if a tumor is not detectable either on grayscale US or CEUS, there is still the possibility of conducting RFA, since we can estimate the approximate location of the tumor using the US fusion imaging system. In particular, a GPS function installed in Volume Navigation System is very helpful in locating such HCCs. When GPS markers are indicated on the target on the reference images, corresponding sites are pinpointed on real-time US images [20]. Therefore, the site of the targeted tumor can be easily identified, even if it is undetectable on US (fig. 1). Thus, we could successfully conduct RFA on 5 HCCs undetectable on grayscale US. In this way, it has become possible to perform RFA for HCCs with poor conspicuity on grayscale US since the introduction of the US fusion imaging system.

As for reference images in the US fusion imaging system, the hepatobiliary phase of Gd-EOB-enhanced MRI was most frequently used and considered most optimal. One of the reasons is that it has the highest sensitivity for detecting HCC [9, 10, 22–24, 33] as described above, and another is the clear depiction of tumors and surrounding intrahepatic landmarks [30], which makes the positional registration accurate and easy.

Conclusion

The usefulness of the US fusion imaging system for RFA of HCC was verified in this study. Although some limitations are still left in terms of the accuracy and the long-term prognosis has not been fully investigated yet, it has greatly extended the indication of RFA. The US fusion imaging system is certainly a valuable tool which enables us to take advantage of the benefits of early diagnosis and treatment of HCC.

Disclosure Statement

The authors declare that no financial or other conflict of interest exists in relation to the content of the article.

References

1 Jemal A, Bray F, Center MM, Ferlay J, Ward E, Forman D: Global cancer statistics. CA Cancer J Clin 2011;61:69–90.

2 Imai Y, Kawata S, Tamura S, Yabuuchi I, Noda S, Inada M, Maeda Y, Shirai Y, Fukuzaki T, Kaji I, Ishikawa H, Matsuda Y, Nishikawa M, Seki K, Matsuzawa Y: Relation of interferon therapy and hepatocellular carcinoma in patients with chronic hepatitis C. Ann Intern Med 1998;129:94–99.

3 Kudo M, Izumi N, Kokudo N, Matsui O, Sakamoto M, Nakashima O, Kojiro M, Makuuchi M, HCC Expert Panel of Japan Society of Hepatology: Management of hepatocellular carcinoma in Japan: Consensus-Based Clinical Practice Guidelines proposed by the Japan Society of Hepatology (JSH) 2010 updated version. Dig Dis 2011;29:339–364.

4 European Association for the Study of the Liver, European Organisation for Research and Treatment of Cancer: EASL-EORTC clinical practice guidelines: management of hepatocellular carcinoma. J Hepatol 2012;56:908–943.

5 Bruix J, Sherman M, American Association for the Study of Liver Diseases: Management of hepatocellular carcinoma: an update. Hepatology 2011;53:1020–1022.

6 Ansari D, Andersson R: Radiofrequency ablation or percutaneous ethanol injection for the treatment of liver tumors. World J Gastroenterol 2012;18:1003–1008.

7 Lencioni R, Crocetti L: Local-regional treatment of hepatocellular carcinoma. Radiology 2012;262:43–58.

8 Murakami T, Imai Y, Okada M, Hyodo T, Lee WJ, Kim MJ, Kim T, Choi BI: Ultrasonography, computed tomography and magnetic resonance imaging of hepatocellular carcinoma: toward improved treatment decisions. Oncology 2011;81;86–99.

9 Kogita S, Imai Y, Okada M, Kim T, Onishi H, Takamura M, Fukuda K, Igura T, Sawai Y, Morimoto O, Hori M, Nagano H, Wakasa K, Hayashi N, Murakami T: Gd-EOB-DTPA-enhanced magnetic resonance images of hepatocellular carcinoma: correlation with histological grading and portal blood flow. Eur Radiol 2010;20:2405–2413.

10 Onishi H, Kim T, Imai Y, Hori M, Nagano H, Nakaya Y, Tsuboyama T, Nakamoto A, Tatsumi M, Kumano S, Okada M, Takamura M, Wakasa K, Tomiyama N, Murakami T: Hypervascular hepatocellular carcinomas: detection with gadoxetate disodium-enhanced MR imaging and multiphasic multidetector CT. Eur Radiol 2012;22:845–854.

11 Kudo M, Hatanaka K, Kumada T, Toyoda H, Tada T: Double-contrast ultrasound: a novel surveillance tool for hepatocellular carcinoma. Am J Gastroenterol 2011;106:368–370.

12 Lee JM, Yoon JH, Joo I, Woo HS: Recent advances in CT and MR imaging for evaluation of hepatocellular carcinoma. Liver Cancer 2012;1:22–40.

13 Ricke J, Seidensticker M, Mohnike K: Non-invasive diagnosis of hepatocellular carcinoma in cirrhotic liver: current guidelines and future prospects for radiological imaging. Liver Cancer 2012;1:51–58.

14 Bota S, Piscaglia F, Marinelli S, Pecorelli A, Terzi E, Bolondi L: Comparison of international guidelines for non-invasive diagnosis of hepatocellular carcinoma. Liver Cancer, in press.

15 Kim YJ, Lee MW, Park HS: Small hepatocellular carcinomas: ultrasonography guided percutaneous radiofrequency ablation. Abdom Imaging 2012, E-pub ahead of print.
16 Nakai M, Sato M, Sahara S, Takasaka I, Kawai N, Minamiguchi H, Tanihata H, Kimura M, Takeuchi N: Radiofrequency ablation assisted by real-time virtual sonography and CT for hepatocellular carcinoma undetectable by conventional sonography. Cardiovasc Intervent Radiol 2009;32:62–69.
17 Kunishi Y, Numata K, Morimoto M, Okada M, Kaneko T, Maeda S, Tanaka K: Efficacy of fusion imaging combining sonography and hepatobiliary phase MRI with Gd-EOB-DTPA to detect small hepatocellular carcinoma. AJR Am J Roentgenol 2012;198:106–114.
18 International Consensus Group for Hepatocellular Neoplasia: Pathologic diagnosis of early hepatocellular carcinoma: a report of the international consensus group for hepatocellular neoplasia. Hepatology 2009;49: 658–664.
19 Imai Y, Murakami T, Yoshida S, Nishikawa M, Ohsawa M, Tokunaga K, Murata M, Shibata K, Zushi S, Kurokawa M, Yonezawa T, Kawata S, Takamura M, Nagano H, Sakon M, Monden M, Wakasa K, Nakamura H: Superparamagnetic iron oxide-enhanced magnetic resonance images of hepatocellular carcinoma: correlation with histological grading. Hepatology 2000;32:205–212.
20 Makino Y, Imai Y, Igura T, Ohama H, Kogita S, Sawai Y, Fukuda K, Ohashi H, Murakami T: Usefulness of the multimodality fusion imaging for the diagnosis and treatment of hepatocellular carcinoma. Dig Dis, in press.
21 Lee MW, Rhim H, Cha DI, Kim YJ, Choi D, Kim YS, Lim HK: Percutaneous radiofrequency ablation of hepatocellular carcinoma: fusion imaging guidance for management of lesions with poor conspicuity at conventional sonography. AJR Am J Roentgenol 2012;198:1438–1444.
22 Di Martino M, Marin D, Guerrisi A, Baski M, Galati F, Rossi M, Brozzetti S, Masciangelo R, Passariello R, Catalano C: Intraindividual comparison of gadoxetate disodium-enhanced MR imaging and 64-section multidetector CT in the detection of hepatocellular carcinoma in patients with cirrhosis. Radiology 2010;256:806–816.
23 Sano K, Ichikawa T, Motosugi U, Sou H, Muhi AM, Matsuda M, Nakano M, Sakamoto M, Nakazawa T, Asakawa M, Fujii H, Kitamura T, Enomoto N, Araki T: Imaging study of early hepatocellular carcinoma: usefulness of gadoxetic acid-enhanced MR Imaging. Radiology 2011;261:834–844.
24 Inoue T, Kudo M, Komuta M, Hayaishi S, Ueda T, Takita M, Kitai S, Hatanaka K, Yada N, Hagiwara S, Chung H, Sakurai T, Ueshima K, Sakamoto M, Maenishi O, Hyodo T, Okada M, Kumano S, Murakami T: Assessment of Gd-EOB-DTPA-enhanced MRI for HCC and dysplastic nodules and comparison of detection sensitivity versus MDCT. J Gastroenterol 2012;47:1036–1047.
25 Komorizono Y, Oketani M, Sako K, Yamasaki N, Shibatou T, Maeda M, Kohara K, Shigenobu S, Ishibashi K, Arima T: Risk factors for local recurrence of small hepatocellular carcinoma tumors after a single session, single application of percutaneous radiofrequency ablation. Cancer 2003;97: 1253–1262.
26 Lee MW, Kim YJ, Park HS, Yu NC, Jung SI, Ko SY, Jeon HJ: Targeted sonography for small hepatocellular carcinoma discovered by CT or MRI: factors affecting sonographic detection. AJR 2010;194:396–400.
27 Kim PN, Choi D, Rhim H, Rha SE, Hong HP, Lee J, Choi JI, Kim JW, Seo JW, Lee EJ, Lim HK: Planning ultrasound for percutaneous radiofrequency ablation to treat small (≤3 cm) hepatocellular carcinomas detected on computed tomography or magnetic resonance imaging: a multicenter prospective study to assess factors affecting ultrasound visibility. J Vasc Interv Radiol 2012;23:627–634.
28 Mita K, Kim SR, Kudo M, Imoto S, Nakajima T, Ando K, Fukuda K, Matsuoka T, Maekawa Y, Hayashi Y: Diagnostic sensitivity of imaging modalities for hepatocellular carcinoma smaller than 2 cm. World J Gastroenterol 2010;16:4187–4192.
29 Minami Y, Kudo M: Review of dynamic contrast-enhanced ultrasound guidance in ablation therapy for hepatocellular carcinoma. World J Gastroenterol 2011;17:4952–4259.
30 Numata K, Luo W, Morimoto M, Kondo M, Kunishi Y, Sasaki T, Nozaki A, Tanaka K: Contrast enhanced ultrasound of hepatocellular carcinoma. World J Radiol 2010;2:68–82.
31 Wong GL, Xu HX, Xie XY: Detection of focal liver lesions in cirrhotic liver using contrast-enhanced ultrasound. World J Radiol 2009; 1:25–36.
32 Arita J, Hasegawa K, Takahashi M, Hata S, Shindoh J, Sugawara Y, Kokudo N: Correlation between contrast-enhanced intraoperative ultrasound using Sonazoid and histologic grade of resected hepatocellular carcinoma. AJR Am J Roentgenol 2011;196: 1314–1321.
33 Golfieri R, Renzulli M, Lucidi V, Corcioni B, Trevisani F, Bolondi L: Contribution of the hepatobiliary phase of Gd-EOB-DTPA-enhanced MRI to Dynamic MRI in the detection of hypovascular small (≤2 cm) HCC in cirrhosis. Eur Radiol 2011;21:1233–1242.

Oncology

Oncology 2013;84(suppl 1):51–57
DOI: 10.1159/000345890

Published online: February 20, 2013

Usefulness of Contrast-Enhanced Ultrasonography to Evaluate the Post-Treatment Responses of Radiofrequency Ablation for Hepatocellular Carcinoma: Comparison with Dynamic CT

Tatsuo Inoue Masatoshi Kudo Kinuyo Hatanaka Tadaaki Arizumi Masahiro Takita Satoshi Kitai Norihisa Yada Satoru Hagiwara Yasunori Minami Toshiharu Sakurai Kazuomi Ueshima Naoshi Nishida

Division of Gastroenterology and Hepatology, Department of Internal Medicine, Kinki University Faculty of Medicine, Osakasayama, Japan

Key Words

Hepatocellular carcinoma · Radiofrequency ablation · Treatment response · Contrast-enhanced ultrasonography · Defect-reperfusion imaging

Abstract

Objective: Contrast-enhanced ultrasonography (CEUS) with Sonazoid® and dynamic computed tomography (CT) were used to evaluate radiofrequency ablation (RFA) for hepatocellular carcinoma (HCC). Local recurrence rate was used as the gold standard of evaluation. ***Methods:*** From January 2007 to December 2011, 86 HCCs from 70 patients were treated with RFA. CEUS with Sonazoid and dynamic CT were then used to evaluate the effect of RFA. For CEUS and dynamic CT, effects were classified as follows: (1) complete ablated response with safety margin >5 mm (CRSM+); (2) complete ablated response but with safety margin <5 mm (CRSM–); (3) incomplete, residual tumor detected after treatment. ***Results:*** CEUS judged 33 cases as CRSM+, while dynamic CT identified 49 cases. None of these 33 cases from the CEUS group had local recurrences, while dynamic CT had 1 case. CEUS judged 49 cases as CRSM–, compared to 34 cases with dynamic CT. Of these, 9 cases of CEUS and 8 cases of dynamic CT showed local recurrences. Two cases diagnosed as 'incomplete' by CEUS and dynamic CT had recurrences within 1 year. ***Conclusion:*** CEUS can be used to assess the efficacy of RFA for HCC, with the potential to reduce the number of CT scans required for confirmation.

Introduction

Hepatocellular carcinoma (HCC) ranks worldwide as the sixth most common cancer and as the third most common cause of cancer deaths. For patients with HCC, percutaneous radiofrequency ablation (RFA) has recently been established as a promising and safe technique [1–4]. RFA has steadily become a first-line ablative procedure for small- to intermediate-sized (3 cm) HCCs at many centers. It has a primary effectiveness rate of 88–99% in treating HCC [5–9]. Dynamic computed tomography (CT) is commonly used for evaluating the response of HCC after RFA [10–12]. However, the use of dynamic CT is prohibited for patients with renal dysfunction and iodine allergy. Another concern for patients is to minimize the exposure to radiation.

KARGER

Fax +41 61 306 12 34
E-Mail karger@karger.com
www.karger.com

0030–2414/13/0847–0051$38.00/0

Accessible online at:
www.karger.com/ocl

Masatoshi Kudo, MD, PhD
Division of Gastroenterology and Hepatology, Department of Internal Medicine
Kinki University Faculty of Medicine
377-2 Ohno-Higashi, Osakasayama, Osaka 589-8511 (Japan)
E-Mail m-kudo@med.kindai.ac.jp

Sonazoid® (Daiichi-Sankyo, Tokyo, Japan; GE Healthcare, Milwaukee, Wisc., USA), a lipid-stabilized suspension of perfluorobutane gas microbubbles was approved exclusively in Japan in January 2007. It facilitates obtaining a real-time blood flow image in addition to a stable Kupffer phase [13]. Sonazoid is a second-generation contrast agent possessing superior qualities over other agents that enabled the acquisition of a good real-time vascular image and a very stable Kupffer-phase image lasting up to 120 min after injection [14, 15]. Defect reperfusion imaging is an innovative technique by which the arterial blood flow can be demonstrated in nodules that show a defect in the Kupffer phase owing to the stability of the Kupffer image with Sonazoid. This is a unique property of Sonazoid and dual phase contrast ultrasound is now a breakthrough in the diagnostic imaging of HCC [14, 16]. By using defect reperfusion imaging in the assessment of RFA, an ablated area can be visualized clearly. Furthermore, a residual nodule or recurrence can be diagnosed by assuming that the defect reinjection sign was positive when arterial vascularity was noted inside a Kupffer defect area. In the present study, the defect reperfusion imaging procedure with Sonazoid was used in assessing the response to RFA. The results were then compared with dynamic CT.

Materials and Methods

Patients

From January 2007 to December 2011, 70 patients (41 males and 29 females; age range 52–83 years) with HCC underwent RFA. Sixty-two patients had cirrhosis (56 with Child-Pugh A and 6 with Child-Pugh B), and 8 patients had chronic hepatitis. Baseline features of the study population are summarized in table 1. All patients met the following criteria for treatment with percutaneous RFA: percutaneous accessibility of the tumor; absence of portal venous and extrahepatic metastases; prothrombin time ratio >50%; total bilirubin concentration <3.0 mg/dl, and platelet count >50,000/μl. Patients were excluded if they had an excessive bleeding tendency (platelet count <50,000/μl or prothrombin activity <50%) or refractory ascites. The study was performed according to the guidelines of the Helsinki Declaration and was approved by our institution's ethics committee. Written, fully informed consent was obtained from each patient before treatment.

Diagnosis of HCC

The diagnosis of HCC was made by the presence of typical tumor features, such as hyperattenuations in the arterial phase and hypoattenuations in the portal phase, using dynamic CT with 64 detectors (LightSpeed VCT; GE Healthcare) [17, 18]. The median diameter of HCC was 16.5 ± 7.1 mm on B-mode ultrasonography (US). All patients underwent dynamic CT during the month before RFA.

Table 1. Baseline features of study population

Patients, n	70
Tumors, n	86
Mean age, years	70.7 ± 7.1
Sex (male/female)	41/29
Size of tumors, cm	16.5 ± 7.1
Follow-up, days	873 ± 426
Child-Pugh (A/B/C)	64/6/0

RFA Technique

All RFAs were performed percutaneously by experienced hepatologists, each of whom had more than 5 years of experience in US-guided interventional procedures and RFA. The treatments were performed under local anesthesia and conscious sedation. Patients were treated with a cooled-tip needle RFA system (Cool-tip, Covidien, Dublin, Ireland), which is a 480-kHz alternative current generator that can produce a maximum power of 180 W through a 17-gauge monopolar cooled-tip needle electrode. A single 2-cm exposed tip was selected for nodules <2 cm in diameter and a single 3-cm exposed tip for larger nodules.

Evaluation of Post-Treatment Effect of RFA

Evaluation of the Effect of RFA Using Contrast-Enhanced US (CEUS). CEUS was performed using a GE LOGIQ 7 ultrasound scanner with a 4.0- or 6.5-MHz convex transducer. The acoustic power of contrast-enhanced harmonic US was set at the default setting with a mechanical index of 0.2; the dynamic range was fixed at 60–65 dB. A single focus point was set at a depth of 10 cm. Data were analyzed and defined by consensus of two hepatologists (T.I., K.H.) who were blinded to the results of evaluation by dynamic CT. In case of discrepancy, the reviewers assessed the saved images together and their findings were re-evaluated to reach an agreement. Defect reperfusion imaging [14, 19] was used to evaluate the Kupffer phase of CEUS with Sonazoid (fig. 1, 2). When the tumor was completely ablated with a safe margin of more than 5 mm, the effectiveness was graded as (CRSM+). When the tumor was completely ablated but with a safe margin less than 5 mm, the effectiveness was graded as (CRSM–). When there were residual tumors (reperfusion areas adjacent to the ablated tumor in the defect reperfusion test), the grading was recorded as 'incomplete', indicative of a residual tumor after treatment. All CEUS studies were performed within 1–3 days of RFA.

Evaluation of Treatment Effect of RFA Using Dynamic CT. Dynamic CT data were analyzed and defined by consensus of two hepatologists (M.K., T.A.) who were blinded to the results of contrast-enhanced US. In case of discrepancy, the reviewers assessed the saved images together and their findings were re-evaluated to reach an agreement. A CT scan with a 5-mm section thickness was performed 1–3 days after RFA to evaluate its effectiveness [1]. When the tumor was completely ablated with a safe margin of more than 5 mm, the effectiveness was graded as CRSM+. When the tumor was completely ablated but with a safe margin less than 5 mm, the effectiveness was graded as (CRSM–). When there were residual tumors (hyperattenuations in the arterial phase and hypoattenuation areas in the portal phase adjacent to the tumor) the grading was recorded as 'incomplete', indicating a residual tumor after treatment.

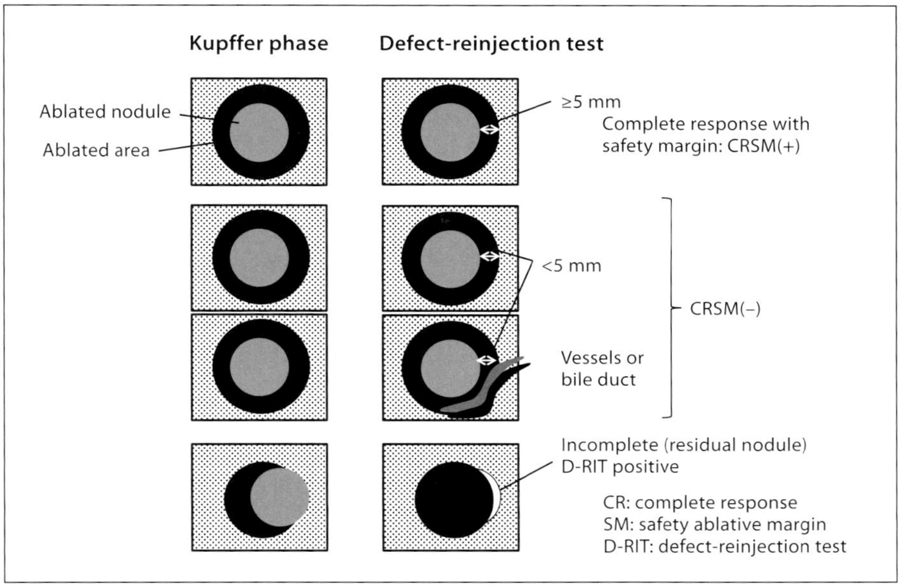

Fig. 1. Evaluation of post-treatment effect of RFA using defect reperfusion test 1. When the ablated tumor was detected on Kupffer-phase image, post-treatment effect was evaluated using the technique shown here. Briefly, in Kupffer phase, the ablated area was observed after reinjection of Sonazoid. If the tumor was completely ablated with adequate safety margin (>5 mm), the therapeutic effect was judged as CRSM(+). If the tumor was ablated without adequate safety margin (<5 mm) or there were some vessels close to tumors within 5 mm, the therapeutic effect was judged as CRSM(–). If there were reperfusion areas on the defect reperfusion test, they were judged as incomplete (residual tumor).

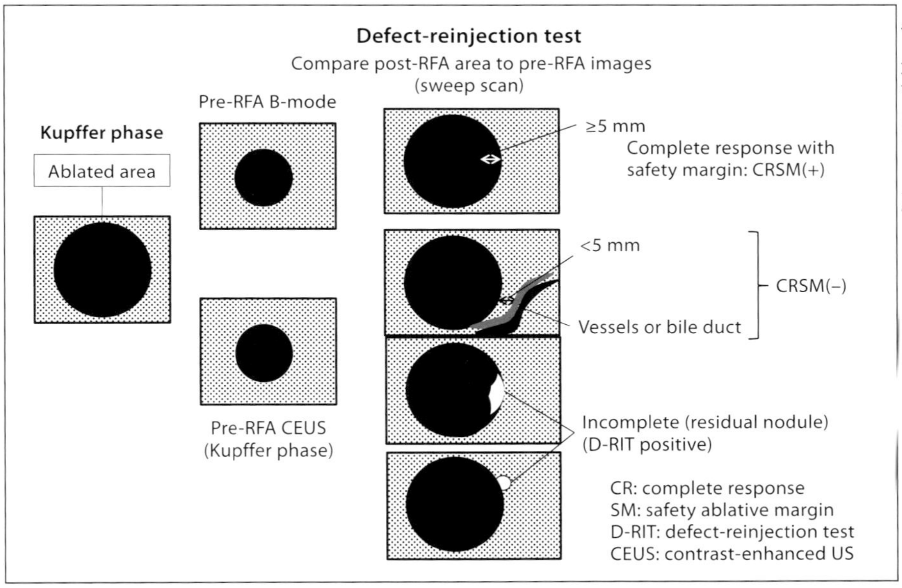

Fig. 2. Evaluation of post-treatment effect of RFA using defect reperfusion test 2. When the ablated tumor cannot be detected on Kupffer-phase image, the safety margin was evaluated by comparing images of pre-B-mode or Kupffer-phase images of HCCs with postablated areas side by side on the US screen.

Assessment of Local Recurrence

Tumor recurrence rates were assessed by performing dynamic CT every 3–4 months after RFA. Local tumor recurrence was defined as the appearance of a viable tumor during follow-up that was contiguous with the zone that had been ablated.

Statistical Analysis

Cumulative incidence of local tumor recurrence was calculated using the Kaplan-Meier test and Fisher's exact test was used to analyze the data. The level of significance was set at $p < 0.05$. All analyses were performed with statistical software (SPSS version 11, SPSS Inc., Chicago, Ill., USA) for Microsoft Windows.

Results

Post-Treatment Evaluation of RFA for HCC Using Each Modality

At the initial evaluation of post-treatment effect of RFA there were 33 and 49 cases judged CRSM+ by CEUS and dynamic CT, respectively. Also, there were 49 and 34 cases judged CRSM– by CEUS and dynamic CT, respectively. CEUS and multidetector CT each judged 3 cases as 'incomplete'. Two cases out of 3 were judged 'incomplete' on both contrast-enhanced US and dynamic CT.

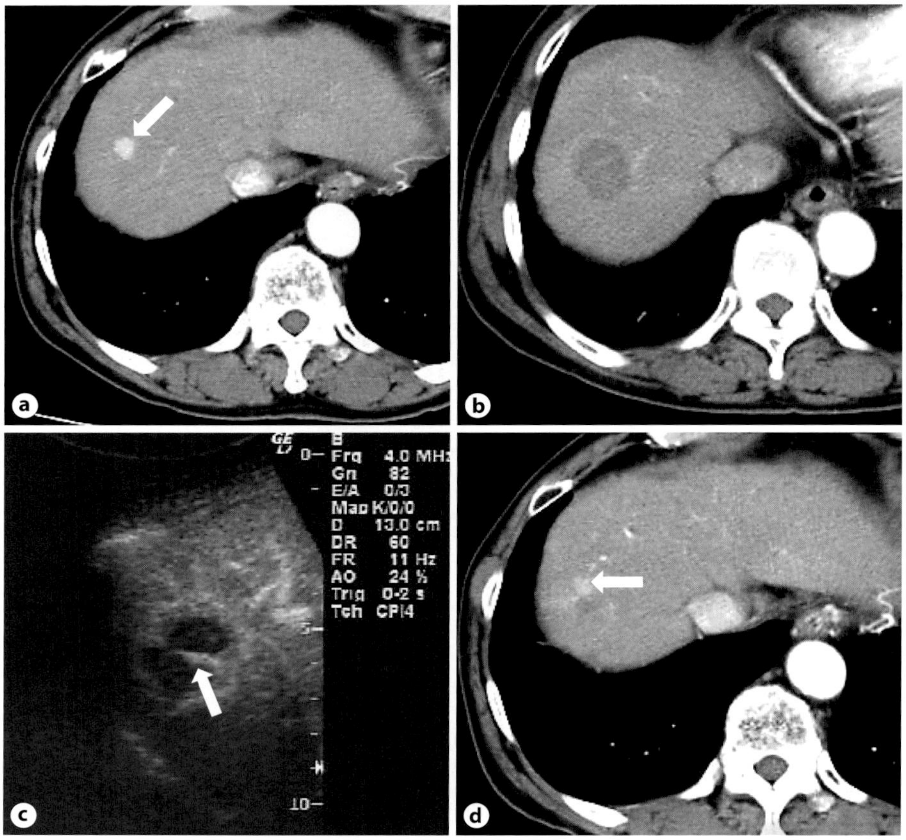

Fig. 3. Case presentation of local tumor recurrence after RFA. **a** A 62-year-old man with a 1.3-cm HCC; Dynamic CT shows a hypervascular tumor (arrow) in segment VIII; RFA was performed on 25th July, 2007. **b** On dynamic CT, the effect of RFA was judged as complete response with a safety margin >5 mm (CRSM+). **c** By using a defect reperfusion test in Kupffer phase, there was a vessel in the ablated area (arrow); the judgment by CEUS was complete response without a safety ablative margin (CRSM–). **d** Local tumor recurrence was observed on 4th June 2008 (arrow).

Table 2. Post-treatment evaluation of RFA for HCC using each modality

Dynamic CT	Contrast-enhanced US			
	CRSM(+)	CRSM(–)	incomplete	N/A
CRSM(+)	30	19	0	0
CRSM(–)	3	29	1	1
Incomplete	0	1	2	0

N/A = Not available.

Table 3. Result of the local recurrence rate according to the therapeutic evaluation of each modality

	Post-treatment evaluation			
	CRSM(+)	CRSM(–)	incomplete	N/A
Dynamic CT	1/49 (2.5%)[1]	8/34 (30%)[1]	3/3	0
Contrast-enhanced US	0/33 (0%)[1]	9/49 (18%)[1]	3/3	0/1

N/A = Not available. [1] Fisher's exact test.

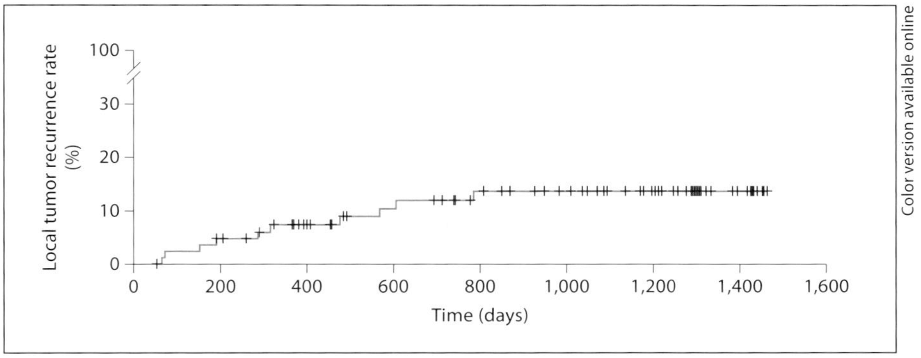

Fig. 4. Cumulative local tumor recurrence rate after RFA of the present study: 9% in 1 year and 12% in 2 years.

One case which could not be evaluated by CEUS was judged as CRSM– by dynamic CT. The consistency of the evaluation result of each modality was 71% (61/86) (table 2).

Local Tumor Recurrence

Two cases were judged 'incomplete' on both contrast-enhanced US and dynamic CT and these were eliminated from the calculation of the cumulative local tumor recurrence rate. Finally, local tumor recurrence was investigated in 84 nodules of 68 patients. Ten of the 84 nodules developed a local tumor recurrence (fig. 3). The cumulative local tumor recurrence rates were 9 and 12% in 1 and 2 years, respectively (fig. 4).

Evaluation of Local Recurrence Rates for Each Modality

Recurrence rates in the CRSM+ and CRSM– groups of dynamic CT were 2.5% (1/49) and 30% (8/34), respectively. Recurrence rates in the CRSM+ and CRSM– groups of CEUS were 0% (0/33) and 18% (9/49), respectively. There were no differences between dynamic CT and CEUS for each of the 3 evaluations, i.e. CRSM+, CRSM– and 'incomplete' (not significant by Fisher's exact test; table 3).

Discussion

Post-treatment responses of percutaneous ethanol injection and RFA for HCC using CEUS have been evaluated in several studies [20–24]. However, precise evaluation was difficult because Doppler US studies with contrast agents were affected by blooming artifacts, poor spatial resolution and low sensitivity to slow flow [20]. Levovist (SH U 508A; Schering AG, Berlin, Germany), was effective only when imaging was performed at high acoustic power using a high mechanical index, but the effect was transient [21, 22]. SonoVue (Bracco, Milan, Italy) is widely available for contrast visualization in Europe and China and is thought to be a truly intravascular, blood-pool contrast agent, with no interstitial equilibrium phase. When parenchyma-specific contrast images can be seen only 3–5 min after the injection, a precise post-treatment evaluation is difficult [23, 24]. Unlike Levovist and SonoVue, Sonazoid has a very stable Kupffer-phase image that may last up to 120 min after its injection. Therefore, in the present study, post-RFA areas were easily detected as perfusion defects in the Kupffer phase. If tumors inside the ablated areas can be detected in the Kupffer phase, safe margins can be clearly seen by using defect reperfusion imaging. Even if tumors cannot be detected in the ablated areas after RFA, safe margins can be evaluated by carefully comparing images of pre-B-mode or Kupffer-phase images of HCCs with postablated areas in the Kupffer phase side by side on the US screen. If arterial perfusion within the defect is demonstrated by the reinjection test of Sonazoid, it can easily define a residual tumor, or if some vessels recognized by the reinjection test are inside ablated areas, the adequacy of the safety margin can be determined. Kim et al. [25] and Nakazawa et al. [26] reported that an ablation zone with a margin of 5 mm or greater was the most important factor for local control of HCC. Therefore, we evaluated the local recurrence rate with or without adequate margins (more than 5 mm). Local recurrence rates between contrast-enhanced US and dynamic CT on each evaluation showed no difference and the consistency of the evaluation result of each modality was 71%. This indicated that CEUS is also useful to evaluate the response of RFA. To date, dynamic CT has been used most frequently to assess the effectiveness of RFA for HCC treatment. However, dynamic CT is prohibited for patients with renal dysfunction and iodine allergy. It is also preferable for the patients to refrain from exposure to radiation. MRI has also been used for evaluating the therapeutic effect of RFA [27, 28]. However, patients who have a heart pacemaker, a metallic foreign body (metal sliver) in the eye or an aneurysm clip in the brain, cannot have an MRI scan because the magnetic field may dislodge the metal. It has been reported that another contrast agent like gadolinium sometimes causes nephrogenic systemic sclerosis [29].

Compared with dynamic CT and MRI [12], Sonazoid enhanced US has none of the risks mentioned above for the patients. Furthermore, CEUS is less expensive than CT and MRI and can be performed numerous times [30, 31].

This study had several limitations. First, it was a retrospective review of HCCs examined by CEUS using Sonazoid and dynamic CT nearly simultaneously after treatment, and there was a bias in the selection of the lesions. Second, the number of evaluated lesions was small. Third, histopathologic findings were not obtained from all patients for the diagnosis of local recurrence. To evaluate the true usefulness of CEUS using Sonazoid for the detection of local recurrence after treatment for HCC, further prospective randomized studies with a larger number of patients are warranted. In conclusion, CEUS with Sonazoid can be used to assess the efficacy of RFA for HCC, with the potential of reducing the number of CT scans required for confirmation.

Disclosure Statement

The authors declare that no conflicts of interests exist.

References

1 Shiina S, Tateishi R, Arano T, Uchino K, Enooku K, Nakagawa H, et al: Radiofrequency ablation for hepatocellular carcinoma: 10-year outcome and prognostic factors. Am J Gastroenterol 2012;107:569–578.

2 Shibata T, Iimuro Y, Yamamoto Y, Maetani Y, Ametani F, Itoh K, et al: Small hepatocellular carcinoma: comparison of radio-frequency ablation and percutaneous microwave coagulation therapy. Radiology 2002; 223:331–337.

3 Wood TF, Rose DM, Chung M, Allegra DP, Foshag LJ, Bilchik AJ: Radiofrequency ablation of 231 unresectable hepatic tumors: indications, limitations, and complications. Ann Surg Oncol 2000;7:593–600.

4 Livraghi T, Goldberg SN, Lazzaroni S, Meloni F, Solbiati L, Gazelle GS: Small hepatocellular carcinoma: treatment with radio-frequency ablation versus ethanol injection. Radiology 1999;210:655–661.

5 Tateishi R, Shiina S, Teratani T, Obi S, Sato S, Koike Y, et al: Percutaneous radiofrequency ablation for hepatocellular carcinoma: an analysis of 1,000 cases. Cancer 2005;103: 1201–1209.

6 Teratani T, Yoshida H, Shiina S, Obi S, Sato S, Tateishi R, et al: Radiofrequency ablation for hepatocellular carcinoma in so-called high-risk locations. Hepatology 2006;43: 1101–1108.

7 Camma C, Di Marco V, Orlando A, Sandonato L, Casaril A, Parisi P, et al: Treatment of hepatocellular carcinoma in compensated cirrhosis with radio-frequency thermal ablation (RFTA): a prospective study. J Hepatol 2005;42:535–540.

8 Lencioni RA, Allgaier HP, Cioni D, Olschewski M, Deibert P, Crocetti L, et al: Small hepatocellular carcinoma in cirrhosis: randomized comparison of radio-frequency thermal ablation versus percutaneous ethanol injection. Radiology 2003;228:235–240.

9 Tiong L, Maddern GJ: Systematic review and meta-analysis of survival and disease recurrence after radiofrequency ablation for hepatocellular carcinoma. Br J Surg 2011;98: 1210–1224.

10 Lim HK, Choi D, Lee WJ, Kim SH, Lee SJ, Jang HJ, et al: Hepatocellular carcinoma treated with percutaneous radio-frequency ablation: evaluation with follow-up multiphase helical CT. Radiology 2001;221:447–454.

11 Chopra S, Dodd GD 3rd, Chintapalli KN, Leyendecker JR, Karahan OI, Rhim H: Tumor recurrence after radiofrequency thermal ablation of hepatic tumors: spectrum of findings on dual-phase contrast-enhanced CT. AJR Am J Roentgenol 2001;177:381–387.

12 Lee JM, Yoon JH, Joo I, Woo HS: Rencet advances in CT and MR imaging for evaluation of hepatocellular carcinoma. Liver Cancer 2012;1:22–40.

13 Halpern EJ, McCue PA, Aksnes AK, Hagen EK, Frauscher F, Gomella LG: Contrast-enhanced US of the prostate with Sonazoid: comparison with whole-mount prostatectomy specimens in 12 patients. Radiology 2002;222:361–366.

14 Kudo M, Hatanaka K, Kumada T, Toyoda H, Tada T: Double-contrast ultrasound: a novel surveillance tool for hepatocellular carcinoma. Am J Gastroenterol 2011;106:368–370.

15 Hatanaka K, Kudo M, Minami Y, Maekawa K: Sonazoid-enhanced ultrasonography for diagnosis of hepatic malignancies: comparison with contrast-enhanced CT. Oncology 2008;75(suppl 1):42–47.

16 Kudo M, Hatanaka K, Maekawa K: Newly developed novel ultrasound technique, defect reperfusion ultrasound imaging, using sonazoid in the management of hepatocellular carcinoma. Oncology 2010;78(suppl 1): 40–45.

17 Kudo M, Okanoue T, Japan Society of Hepatology: Management of hepatocellular carcinoma in Japan: consensus-based clinical practice manual proposed by the Japan Society of Hepatology. Oncology 2007;72(suppl 1):2–15.

18 Bruix J, Sherman M: Management of hepatocellular carcinoma: an update. Hepatology 2011;53:1020–1022.

19 Kudo M, Hatanaka K, Maekawa K: Defect reperfusion imaging, a newly developed novel technology using Sonazoid in the treatment of hepatocellular carcinoma. J Med Ultrasound 2008;16:169–175.

20 Bartolozzi C, Lencioni R, Ricci P, Paolicchi A, Rossi P, Passariello R: Hepatocellular carcinoma treatment with percutaneous ethanol injection: evaluation with contrast-enhanced color Doppler US. Radiology 1998; 209:387–393.

21 Ding H, Kudo M, Onda H, Suetomi Y, Minami Y, Chung H, et al: Evaluation of post-treatment response of hepatocellular carcinoma with contrast-enhanced coded phase-inversion harmonic US: comparison with dynamic CT. Radiology 2001;221:721–730.

22 Ding H, Kudo M, Onda H, Suetomi Y, Minami Y, Maekawa K: Contrast-enhanced subtraction harmonic sonography for evaluating treatment response in patients with hepatocellular carcinoma. AJR Am J Roentgenol 2001;176:661–666.
23 Frieser M, Kiesel J, Lindner A, Bernatik T, Haensler JM, Janka R, et al: Efficacy of contrast-enhanced US versus CT or MRI for the therapeutic control of percutaneous radiofrequency ablation in the case of hepatic malignancies. Ultraschall Med 2011;32:148–153.
24 Ricci P, Cantisani V, Drudi F, Pagliara E, Bezzi M, Meloni F, et al: Is contrast-enhanced US alternative to spiral CT in the assessment of treatment outcome of radiofrequency ablation in hepatocellular carcinoma? Ultraschall Med 2009;30:252–258.
25 Kim YS, Rhim H, Cho OK, Koh BH, Kim Y: Intrahepatic recurrence after percutaneous radiofrequency ablation of hepatocellular carcinoma: analysis of the pattern and risk factors. Eur J Radiol 2006;59:432–441.
26 Nakazawa T, Kokubu S, Shibuya A, Ono K, Watanabe M, Hidaka H, et al: Radiofrequency ablation of hepatocellular carcinoma: correlation between local tumor progression after ablation and ablative margin. AJR Am J Roentgenol 2007;188:480–448.
27 Tokunaga S, Koda M, Matono T, Sugihara T, Nagahara T, Ueki M, et al: Assessment of ablative margin by MRI with ferucarbotran in radiofrequency ablation for liver cancer: comparison with enhanced CT. Br J Radiol 2012;85:745–752.
28 Koda M, Tokunaga S, Miyoshi K, Kishina M, Fujise Y, Kato J, et al: Assessment of ablative margin by unenhanced magnetic resonance imaging after radiofrequency ablation for hepatocellular carcinoma. Eur J Radiol 2012; 81:2730–2736.
29 Grobner T, Prischl FC: Gadolinium and nephrogenic systemic fibrosis. Kidney Int 2007;72:260–264.
30 Joo I, Choi BI: New paradigm for management of hepatocellular carcinoma by imaging. Liver Cancer 2012;1:94–109.
31 Salvatore V, Bolondi L: Clinical impact of ultrasound-related techniques in the diagnosis of focal liver lesions. Liver Cancer, 2012;1: 238–246.

Oncology

Oncology 2013;84(suppl 1):58–63
DOI: 10.1159/000345891

Published online: February 20, 2013

Therapeutic Response Assessment of Transcatheter Arterial Chemoembolization for Hepatocellular Carcinoma: Ultrasonography, CT and MR Imaging

Yasunori Minami Masatoshi Kudo

Department of Gastroenterology and Hepatology, Kinki University Faculty of Medicine, Osakasayama, Japan

Key Words

Computed tomography · Hepatocellular carcinoma · Magnetic resonance imaging · Transcatheter arterial chemoembolization · Ultrasonography

Abstract

Two randomized controlled trials identified that transcatheter arterial chemoembolization (TACE) for hepatocellular carcinoma (HCC) shows a significant survival benefit compared with controls, after a long-term controversy. Thus, TACE is the current standard of care for patients presenting with multinodular HCC. Monitoring tumor response to TACE is part of the clinical management of HCC patients. Imaging, including ultrasonography, computed tomography and magnetic resonance imaging, has an important role in assessing therapeutic effects earlier and more objectively. Imaging assessment needs to detect not only a reduction in overall tumor load but also a reduction in viable tumor. Here, we give an overview of the current status of the imaging assessment of HCC response to TACE.

Introduction

The primary goal of cancer treatment is to produce a complete and sustained remission. Monitoring tumor response to therapy is part of the clinical management of cancer patients. Imaging is generally used to assess therapeutic effects earlier and more objectively.

Hepatocellular carcinoma (HCC) is a main leading cause of cancer-related death worldwide [1–4]. HCC may also develop in more than one site in the liver and may grow into multiple tumors. In addition, in a high proportion of cases the disease recurs after radical therapy. Transcatheter arterial chemoembolization (TACE) is the current standard of care for patients presenting with multinodular HCC and relatively preserved liver function, absence of cancer-related symptoms, and no evidence of vascular invasion or extrahepatic spread [5–10]. In 2002, two randomized controlled trials [11–14] identified that TACE showed a significant survival benefit compared with controls after a long-term controversy. TACE has often been performed repeatedly during effective monitoring [15]. However, repetitive TACE treatments might reduce liver function and induce stenosis of the hepatic artery. Furthermore, repetitive TACE treatments can become less effective in patients with relapsed HCC. These cases are considered TACE-refractory in clinical practice [16–18]. It is essential to assess tumor response accurately in order to discontinue ineffective therapies and avoid complications caused by tumor progression. Imaging, including ultrasonography (US), computed tomography (CT) and magnetic resonance imaging (MRI) [19], has an important role in assessing the effectiveness of tumor response of HCC. Therefore, we need to understand the characteristics of each imag-

Masatoshi Kudo, MD, PhD
Division of Gastroenterology and Hepatology, Department of Internal Medicine
Kinki University Faculty of Medicine
377-2 Ohno-Higashi, Osakasayama, Osaka 589-8511 (Japan)
E-Mail m-kudo@med.kindai.ac.jp

ing modality for reading images. In this review, we focus our discussion on the imaging assessment of HCC response to TACE.

Principle of Tumor Response Assessment to TACE for HCC

Tumor shrinkage after therapy is only one parameter affecting patient survival. Conventional methods for response assessment, such as the World Health Organization (WHO) criteria and the Response Evaluation Criteria In Solid Tumors (RECIST), have limited predictive value in HCC patients treated with TACE [20–22]. TACE induces direct tumor necrosis and its anticancer efficacy is not paralleled by a reduction in overall tumor load but rather by a reduction in viable tumor, as recognized by contrast-enhanced radiologic imaging [21, 22]. The guidelines state that assessment of response in HCC should be based on performing contrast-enhanced imaging 1 month after initial treatment and at least every 3 months during follow-up [22, 23]. These criteria rely only on tumor shrinkage as a measure of antitumor activity.

Imaging

Computed Tomography

Recently, drug-eluting beads have provided an attractive alternative to iodized oil-based regimens. However, conventional TACE with administration of an anticancer agent-in-oil emulsion followed by embolic agents has been the most popular technique. Lipiodol (Lipiodol Ultrafluide, Laboratoire Guerbet, Aulnay-Sous-Bois, France) is an oily contrast medium in radiography, and Lipiodol accumulation in the tumor can be regarded as representing a necrotic area [24, 25]. Therefore, CT is commonly used as the standard imaging technique for evaluating the therapeutic response in patients with HCC after TACE (table 1) [26–38].

The accumulation pattern of Lipiodol observed on CT can be classified, and the pattern and distribution of Lipiodol in the tumor are useful for assessing the therapeutic effects of TACE. A greater amount of accumulation of Lipiodol within a tumor indicates a greater area of necrosis. During follow-up, the focal defect or washout of Lipiodol in the mass with the contrast-enhanced area suggests the presence of a viable tumor and that additional treatment is needed. However, Lipiodol can be more difficult to assess on CT because accumulation of Lipiodol in tumors can mask the enhancement of a residual tumor. At least a few weeks are required to evaluate whether Lipiodol accumulation corresponds to the necrotic area on CT because Lipiodol gradually washes out of the viable area in the tumor [25]. Thus, it is considered that early assessment of response of TACE is difficult on contrast-enhanced CT.

Recent developments in flat panel detector technology and rotational angiography techniques can provide 3D imaging information that offers a quality similar to that of CT images. Several studies have shown that cone-beam CT angiography can be extremely helpful during TACE [39–42]. Cone-beam CT would potentially be a convenient tool for very early assessment of response by Lipiodol retention in HCCs immediately after TACE [43].

Ultrasonography

A recent advance in US imaging is the development of microbubble contrast agents, which consist of a gas core that is encapsulated by a shell constructed of a lipid monolayer or cross-linked albumin. Each bubble acts as a harmonic oscillator and contrast-enhanced echo signals contain significant energy components at higher harmonics, while tissue echoes do not. With the use of a contrast agent, contrast harmonic imaging possesses not only a very high sensitivity to the contrast agent but also a high spatial resolution, and can depict signals from microbubbles in very slow flow without Doppler-related artifacts. Consequently, it could be a more accurate way to demonstrate residual viable tumor flow in HCC after therapy. Several researchers have reported that contrast harmonic imaging is a useful tool for assessing vascularity in comparison with contrast-enhanced CT because the tumor vascularity depiction is not affected by Lipiodol accumulation (table 2) [44–52]. Residual tumor blood flow on contrast-enhanced US performed within days to 2 weeks after TACE could be predictive of tumor outcome as an early assessment of response to TACE. Use of contrast-enhanced US permits the proper selection of patients who would benefit from additional focal therapy after TACE earlier, as well as helping to guide focal ablation to the viable portion of HCC [46, 49]. However, contrast-enhanced US has technical limitations imposed by body habitus and the difficulty involved in the accessibility to lesions near the hemidiaphragm and to lesions in some small or diseased livers. Additionally, contrast-enhanced US examinations used to be performed on a solitary mass or on a dominant mass in patients with multiple lesions.

Magnetic Resonance Imaging

MRI provides better contrast between the different soft tissues and higher spatial resolution with sensitivity

Table 1. Assessment of treatment response to TAE/TACE using CT

First author, year	n (patients/ nodules)	Mean tumor size, cm	Procedure	Assessment of response
Takayasu, 1984 [26]	18/ND	ND	TAE	Contrast-enhanced area
Furui, 1984 [27]	50/65	ND	TAE	Contrast-enhanced area
Matsuo, 1993 [28]	12/ND	ND	Lip-TACE	Lipiodol uptake
Nishimine, 1994 [29]	98/ND	ND	Lip-TACE	Lipiodol uptake
Tsushima, 1998 [30]	22/ND	ND	Lip-TACE	Lipiodol uptake + contrast-enhanced area
Ernst, 1999 [31]	160/ND	ND	Lip-TACE	Lipiodol uptake only
Sumi, 1999 [32]	45/142	ND	Lip-TACE	Lipiodol uptake + contrast-enhanced area
Okusaka, 2000 [33]	88/ND	ND	Lip-TACE	Lipiodol uptake + contrast-enhanced area
Cioni, 2000 [34]	47/68	4.3	Lip-TACE	Lipiodol uptake + contrast-enhanced area
Katyal, 2000 [35]	57/ND	ND	TACE	Contrast-enhanced area
Kubota, 2001 [36]	54/84	2.2	Lip-TACE	Lipiodol uptake + contrast-enhanced area
Kim, 2002 [37]	54/129	ND	Lip-TACE	Lipiodol uptake + contrast-enhanced area
Ebied, 2003 [38]	72/186	ND	Lip-TACE	Lipiodol uptake + contrast-enhanced area

Lip = Lipiodol; ND = not described; TAE = transcatheter arterial embolization.

Table 2. Assessment of treatment response to TACE: contrast harmonic US versus contrast-enhanced CT

First author, year	n (patients/ nodules)	Mean tumor size, cm	Contrast agent	Viable area detection rate (US/CT), %
Catalano, 1999 [44]	28/43	3.4	Levovist	91/72
Cioni, 2000 [34]	47/68	4.3	Levovist	88/34
Numata, 2001 [45]	29/39	ND	Levovist	92/33
Minami, 2003 [46]	40/44	3.9	Levovist	86/43
Morimoto, 2003 [47]	29/29	ND	Levovist	57/ND
Kim, 2006 [48]	29/29	2.5	Levovist	61/39
Kono, 2007 [49]	33/42	ND	Optison	78/ND
Xia, 2008 [50]	28/43	1.7	Sonazoid	58/40
Schacherer, 2010 [51]	15/15	4.8	SonoVue	93/73

ND = Not described.

Table 3. Assessment of treatment response to TACE: MRI versus CT

First author, year	n (patients/ nodules)	Mean tumor size, cm	Contrast agent	Viable area detection rate (MRI/CT), %
Yamashita, 1993 [53]	37/44	ND	Gd-DTPA	100/ND
Ito, 1995 [54]	13/13	ND	Gd-DTPA	77/ND
Kubota, 2001 [55]	54/84	2.2	Gd-DTPA	100/76
Minami, 2003 [46]	40/44	3.9	Gd-DTPA	50/43
Chen, 2006 [56]	20/20	ND	none (diffusion-weighted MRI)	100/ND
Kubota, 2010 [57]	25/36	2.0	none (diffusion-weighted MRI)	92/92

ND = Not described.

than CT. Recent advances in MRI, including breath-hold 3D imaging and rapid half-Fourier acquisition, allow imaging of the liver in a single breath-hold with a high spatial resolution. Various contrast agents are available to image the liver. A paramagnetic ion, gadolinium-diethylenetriamine pentaacetic acid, is the most commonly used MRI contrast agent; it has an extracellular distribution and behaves similarly to the iodinated contrast agents used in CT. The presence of gadolinium can strongly influence the relaxation properties of nearby protons, leading to changes in tissue contrast. Liver-specific contrast media, such as mangafodipir trisodium (taken up by hepatocytes) and ferrum oxides (taken up by Kupffer cells), demonstrate selective uptake in the liver and are primarily used for lesion detection.

Lipiodol causes variable signal intensity changes on unenhanced MRI, and it is difficult to detect accurately [24]. Enhanced areas in the embolization site on gadolinium-enhanced MRI presumably represent viable tumor (table 3) [53–57] but could also result from post-treatment granulation tissue [58]. In addition, diffusion-weighted MRI is a new kind of functional imaging technology that can explore the random diffusion motion of water molecules in vivo. Diffusion-weighted MRI has been found to be useful for lesion detection with higher accuracy compared with superparamagnetic iron oxide-enhanced MRI [59]. However, diffusion-weighted MRI is known to have limitations such as a relatively poor signal-to-noise ratio and high sensitivity to pulsatile or susceptibility artifacts, degrading the ability to detect lesions. A new quantitative measurement on diffusion-weighted MRI may allow effective evaluation of the efficacy of TACE for HCC and correctly reveal recurrent tumors [56, 57].

Conclusion

Conventional TACE with administration of an anticancer agent-in-oil emulsion followed by embolic agents has been the most popular technique. Imaging, including US, CT and MRI, has an important role in assessing the effectiveness of tumor response of HCC. Imaging assessment needs to detect not only a reduction in overall tumor load, but also a reduction in viable tumor.

CT is commonly used as the standard imaging technique because the accumulation of Lipiodol is observed easily on plain CT. Distribution of Lipiodol in the tumor is useful for assessing the therapeutic effects on CT. However, Lipiodol often makes it difficult to detect the residual tumor on CT because accumulation of intratumoral Lipiodol can mask its enhancement. Contrast-enhanced US is a useful tool for assessing the vascularity in comparison with contrast-enhanced CT because the tumor vascularity depiction is not affected by Lipiodol accumulation. However, US examinations used to be performed on a solitary mass or on a dominant mass in patients with multiple lesions. MRI provides better contrast between the different soft tissues and higher spatial resolution than that of CT. Enhanced areas in the embolization site on gadolinium-enhanced MRI presumably represent viable tumor with high sensitivity but low specificity.

Disclosure Statement

The authors declare that no conflicts of interest exist.

References

1 El-Serag HB: Hepatocellular carcinoma. N Engl J Med 2011;365:1118–1127.
2 Parkin DM, Bray F, Ferlay J, Pisani P: Estimating the world cancer burden: Globocan 2000. Int J Cancer 2001;94:153–156.
3 Altekruse SF, McGlynn KA, Reichman ME: Hepatocellular carcinoma incidence, mortality, and survival trends in the United States from 1975 to 2005. J Clin Oncol 2009;27:1485–1491.
4 Kim DY, Han KH: Epidemiology and surveillance of hepatocellular carcinoma. Liver Cancer 2012;1:2–14.
5 Yamada R, Sato M, Kawabata M, Nakatsuka H, Nakamura K, Takashima S: Hepatic artery embolization in 120 patients with unresectable hepatoma. Radiology 1983;148:397–401.
6 Ohishi H, Uchida H, Yoshimura H, Ohue S, Ueda J, Katsuragi M, Matsuo N, Hosogi Y: Hepatocellular carcinoma detected by iodized oil: use of anticancer agents. Radiology 1985;154:25–29.
7 Takayasu K, Shima Y, Muramatsu Y, Moriyama N, Yamada T, Makuuchi M, Hasegawa H, Hirohashi S: Hepatocellular carcinoma: treatment with intraarterial iodized oil with and without chemotherapeutic agents. Radiology 1987;163:345–351.
8 Matsui O, Kadoya M, Yoshikawa J, Gabata T, Arai K, Demachi H, Miyayama S, Takashima T, Unoura M, Kogayashi K: Small hepatocellular carcinoma: treatment with subsegmental transcatheter arterial embolization. Radiology 1993;188:79–83.
9 Takayasu K: Transarterial chemoembolization for hepatocellular carcinoma over three decades: current progress and perspective. Jpn J Clin Oncol 2012;42:247–255.
10 Lencioni R: Chemoembolization for hepatocellular carcinoma. Semin Oncol 2012;39:503–509.
11 Llovet JM, Real MI, Montaña X, Planas R, Coll S, Aponte J, Ayuso C, Sala M, Muchart J, Solà R, Rodés J, Bruix J, Barcelona Liver Cancer Group: Arterial embolisation or chemoembolisation versus symptomatic treatment in patients with unresectable hepatocellular carcinoma: a randomised controlled trial. Lancet 2002;359:1734–1739.

12 Lo CM, Ngan H, Tso WK, Liu CL, Lam CM, Poon RT, Fan ST, Wong J: Randomized controlled trial of transarterial Lipiodol chemoembolization for unresectable hepatocellular carcinoma. Hepatology 2002;35:1164–1171.
13 Lencioni R: Chemoembolization in patients with hepatocellular carcinoma. Liver Cancer 2012;1:41–50.
14 Lin S, Hoffmann K, Schemmer P: Treatment of hepatocellular carcinoma: a systematic review. Liver Cancer 2012;1:144–158.
15 Ikeda K, Kumada H, Saitoh S, Arase Y, Chayama K: Effect of repeated transcatheter arterial embolization on the survival time in patients with hepatocellular carcinoma: an analysis by the Cox proportional hazard model. Cancer 1991;68:2150–2154.
16 Yamanaka K, Hatano E, Kitamura K, Iida T, Ishii T, Machimito T, Taura K, Yasuchika K, Isoda H, Shibata T, Uemoto S: Early evaluation of transcatheter arterial chemoembolization-refractory hepatocellular carcinoma. J Gastroenterol 2012;47:343–346.
17 Kudo M: Treatment of advanced hepatocellular carcinoma with emphasis on hepatic arterial infusion chemotherapy and molecular targeted therapy. Liver Cancer 2012;1:62–70.
18 Kudo M, Izumi N, Kokudo N, Matsui O, Sakamoto M, Nakashima O, Kojiro M, Makuuchi M: Management of hepatocellular carcinoma in Japan: consensus-based clinical practice guidelines proposed by the Japan Society of Hepatology (JSH) 2010 updated version. Dig Dis 2011;29:339–364.
19 Lee JM, Yoon JH, Joo I, Woo HS: Recent advances in CT and MR imaging for evaluation of hepatocellular carcinoma. Liver Cancer 2012;1:22–40.
20 Forner A, Ayuso C, Varela M, Rimola J, Hessheimer AJ, de Lope CR, Reig M, Bianchi L, Llovet JM, Bruix J: Evaluation of tumor response after locoregional therapies in hepatocellular carcinoma: are response evaluation criteria in solid tumors reliable? Cancer 2009;115:616–623.
21 Takayasu K: Transarterial chemoembolization for hepatocellular carcinoma over three decades: current progress and perspective. Jpn J Clin Oncol 2012;42:247–255.
22 Kudo M, Kubo S, Takayasu K, Sakamoto M, Tanaka M, Ikai I, Furuse J, Nakamura K, Makuuchi M, Liver Cancer Study Group of Japan (Committee for Response Evaluation Criteria in Cancer of the Liver): Response Evaluation Criteria in Cancer of the Liver (RECICL) proposed by the Liver Cancer Study Group of Japan (2009 revised version). Hepatol Res 2010;40:686–692.
23 European Association for the Study of the Liver, European Organization for Research and Treatment of Cancer: EASL-EORTC clinical practice guidelines: management of hepatocellular carcinoma. J Hepatol 2012;56: 908–943.
24 Imaeda T, Yamawaki Y, Seki M, Goto H, Iinuma G, Kanematsu M, Mochizuki R, Doi H, Saji S, Shimokawa K: Lipiodol retention and massive necrosis after Lipiodol-chemoembolization of hepatocellular carcinoma: correlation between computed tomography and histopathology. Cardiovasc Intervent Radiol 1993;16:209–213.
25 Takayasu K, Arii S, Matsuo N, Yoshikawa M, Ryu M, Takasaki K, Sato M, Yamanaka N, Shimamura Y, Ohto M: Comparison of CT findings with resected specimens after chemonmbolization with iodized oil for hepatocellular carcinoma. AJR Am J Roentogenol 2000;175:699–704.
26 Takayasu K, Moriyama N, Muramatsu Y, Suzuki M, Yamada T, Kishi K, Hasagawa H, Okazaki N: Hepatic arterial embolization for hepatocellular carcinoma: comparison of CT scans and resected specimens. Radiology 1984;150:661–665.
27 Furui S, Otomo K, Itai Y, Iio M: Hepatocellular carcinoma treated by transcatheter arterial embolization: progress evaluated by computed tomography. Radiology 1984;150: 773–778.
28 Matsuo N, Uchida H, Nishimine K, Soda S, Oshima M, Nakano H, Nagano N, Nishimura Y, Yoshioka T, Guo Q, et al: Segmental transcatheter hepatic artery chemoembolization with iodized oil for hepatocellular carcinoma: antitumor effect and influence on normal tissue. J Vasc Interv Radiol 1993;4:543–549.
29 Nishimine K, Uchida H, Matsuo N, Sakaguchi H, Hirohashi S, Nishimura Y, Guo Q, Ohishi H, Nagano N, Yoshioka T, et al: Segmental transarterial chemoembolization with Lipiodol mixed with anticancer drugs for nonresectable hepatocellular carcinoma: follow-up CT and therapeutic results. Cancer Chemother Pharmacol 1994;33(suppl):S60–S68.
30 Tsushima Y, Unno Y, Koizumi J, Kusano S: Hepatic perfusion changes after transcatheter arterial embolization (TAE) of hepatocellular carcinoma: measurement by dynamic computed tomography (CT). Dig Dis Sci 1998;43:317–322.
31 Ernst O, Sergent G, Mizrahi D, Delemazure O, Paris JC, L'Herminé C: Treatment of hepatocellular carcinoma by transcatheter arterial chemoembolization: comparison of planned periodic chemoembolization and chemoembolization based on tumor response. AJR Am J Roentgenol 1999;172:59–64.
32 Sumi S, Yamashita Y, Mitsuzaki K, Yamamoto H, Urata J, Nishiharu T, Takahashi M: Power Doppler sonography assessment of tumor recurrence after chemoembolization therapy for hepatocellular carcinoma. AJR Am J Roentgenol 1999;172:67–71.
33 Okusaka T, Okada S, Ueno H, Ikeda M, Yoshimori M, Shimada K, Yamamoto J, Kosuge T, Yamasaki S, Iwata R, Furukawa H, Moriyama N, Sakamoto M, Hirohashi S: Evaluation of the therapeutic effect of transcatheter arterial embolization for hepatocellular carcinoma. Oncology 2000;58:293–299.
34 Cioni D, Lencioni R, Bartolozzi C: Therapeutic effect of transcatheter arterial chemoembolization on hepatocellular carcinoma: evaluation with contrast-enhanced harmonic power Doppler ultrasound. Eur Radiol 2000;10:1570–1575.
35 Katyal S, Oliver JH, Peterson MS, Chang PJ, Baron RL, Carr BI: Prognostic significance of arterial phase CT for prediction of response to transcatheter arterial chemoembolization in unresectable hepatocellular carcinoma: a retrospective analysis. AJR Am J Roentgenol 2000;175:1665–1672.
36 Kubota K, Hisa N, Nishikawa T, Fujiwara Y, Murata Y, Itoh S, Yoshida D, Yoshida S: Evaluation of hepatocellular carcinoma after treatment with transcatheter arterial chemoembolization: comparison of Lipiodol-CT, power Doppler sonography, and dynamic MRI. Abdom Imaging 2001;26:184–190.
37 Kim HC, Kim AY, Han JK, Chung JW, Lee JY, Park JH, Choi BI: Hepatic arterial and portal venous phase helical CT in patients treated with transcatheter arterial chemoembolization for hepatocellular carcinoma: added value of unenhanced images. Radiology 2002;225:773–780.
38 Ebied OM, Federle MP, Carr BI, Pealer KM, Li W, Amesur N, Zajko A: Evaluation of responses to chemoembolization in patients with unresectable hepatocellular carcinoma. Cancer 2003;97:1042–1050.
39 Hirota S, Nakao N, Yamamoto S, Kobayashi K, Maeda H, Ishikura R, Miura K, Sakamoto K, Ueda K, Baba R: Cone-beam CT with flat-panel-detector digital angiography system: early experience in abdominal interventional procedures. Cardiovasc Intervent Radiol 2006;29:1034–1038.
40 Kakeda S, Korogi Y, Ohnari N, Moriya J, Oda N, Nishino K, Miyamoto W: Usefulness of cone-beam volume CT with flat panel detectors in conjunction with catheter angiography for transcatheter arterial embolization. J Vasc Interv Radiol 2007;18:1508–1516.
41 Miyayama S, Yamashiro M, Okuda M, Yoshie Y, Sugimori N, Igarashi S, Nakashima Y, Matsui O: Usefulness of cone-beam computed tomography during ultraselective transcatheter arterial chemoembolization for small hepatocellular carcinomas that cannot be demonstrated on angiography. Cardiovasc Intervent Radiol 2009;32:255–264.
42 Higashihara H, Osuga K, Onishi H, Nakamoto A, Tsuboyama T, Maeda N, Hori M, Kim T, Tomiyama N: Diagnostic accuracy of C-arm CT during selective transcatheter angiography for hepatocellular carcinoma: comparison with intravenous contrast-enhanced, biphasic, dynamic MDCT. Eur Radiol 2012;22:872–879.
43 Jeon UB, Lee JW, Choo KS, Kim CW, Kim S, Lee TH, Jeong YJ, Kang DH: Iodized oil uptake assessment with cone-beam CT in chemoembolization of small hepatocellular carcinomas. World J Gastroenterol 2009;15: 5833–5837.

44 Catalano O, Esposito M, Lobianco R, Cusati B, Altei F, Siani A: Hepatocellular carcinoma treated with chemoembolization: assessment with contrast-enhanced doppler ultrasonography. Cardiovasc Intervent Radiol 1999;22:486–492.
45 Numata K, Tanaka K, Kiba T, Saito S, Isozaki T, Hara K, Morimoto M, Sekihara H, Yonezawa H, Kubota T: Using contrast-enhanced sonography to assess the effectiveness of transcatheter arterial embolization for hepatocellular carcinoma. AJR Am J Roentgenol 2001;176:1199–1205.
46 Minami Y, Kudo M, Kawasaki T, Kitano M, Chung H, Maekawa K, Shiozaki H: Transcatheter arterial chemoembolization of hepatocellular carcinoma: usefulness of coded phase-inversion harmonic sonography. AJR Am J Roentgenol 2003;180:703–708.
47 Morimoto M, Shirato K, Sugimori K, Kokawa A, Tomita N, Saito T, Imada T, Tanaka N, Nozawa A, Numata K, Tanaka K: Contrast-enhanced harmonic gray-scale sonographic-histologic correlation of the therapeutic effects of transcatheter arterial chemoembolization in patients with hepatocellular carcinoma. AJR Am J Roentgenol 2003;181: 65–69.
48 Kim HJ, Kim TK, Kim PN, Kim AY, Ko EY, Kim KW, Sung KB, Ha HK, Kim HC, Lee MG: Assessment of the therapeutic response of hepatocellular carcinoma treated with transcatheter arterial chemoembolization: comparison of contrast-enhanced sonography and 3-phase computed tomography. J Ultrasound Med 2006;25:477–486.
49 Kono Y, Lucidarme O, Choi SH, Rose SC, Hassanein TI, Alpert E, Mattrey RF: Contrast-enhanced ultrasound as a predictor of treatment efficacy within 2 weeks after transarterial chemoembolization of hepatocellular carcinoma. J Vasc Interv Radiol 2007;18:57–65.
50 Xia Y, Kudo M, Minami Y, Hatanaka K, Ueshima K, Chung H, Hagiwara S, Inoue T, Ishikawa E, Kitai S, Takahashi S, Tatsumi C, Ueda T, Hayaishi S, Maekawa K: Response evaluation of transcatheter arterial chemoembolization in hepatocellular carcinomas: the usefulness of sonazoid-enhanced harmonic sonography. Oncology 2008;75(suppl 1):99–105.
51 Schacherer D, Girlich C, Zorger N, Wiest R, Schoelmerich J, Feuerbach S, Jung EM: Sono-hepatic-arteriography (Sono-HA) in the assessment of hepatocellular carcinoma in patients undergoing transcatheter arterial chemoembolization (TACE). Ultraschall Med 2010;31:270–275.
52 Salvatore V, Bolondi L: Clinical impact of ultrasound-related techniques in the diagnosis of focal liver lesions. Liver Cancer, in press.
53 Yamashita Y, Yoshimatsu S, Sumi M, Harada M, Takahashi M: Dynamic MR imaging of hepatoma treated by transcatheter arterial embolization therapy: assessment of treatment effect. Acta Radiol 1993;34:303–308.
54 Ito K, Honjo K, Fujita T, Matsui M, Awaya H, Matsumoto T, Matsunaga N, Nakanishi T: Therapeutic efficacy of transcatheter arterial chemoembolization for hepatocellular carcinoma: MRI and pathology. J Comput Assist Tomogr 1995;19:198–203.
55 Kubota K, Hisa N, Nishikawa T, Fujiwara Y, Murata Y, Itoh S, Yoshida D, Yoshida S: Evaluation of hepatocellular carcinoma after treatment with transcatheter arterial chemoembolization: comparison of Lipiodol-CT, power Doppler sonography, and dynamic MRI. Abdom Imaging 2001;26:184–190.
56 Chen CY, Li CW, Kuo YT, Jaw TS, Wu DK, Jao JC, Hsu JS, Liu GC: Early response of hepatocellular carcinoma to transcatheter arterial chemoembolization: choline levels and MR diffusion constants – initial experience. Radiology 2006;239:448–456.
57 Kubota K, Yamanishi T, Itoh S, Murata Y, Miyatake K, Yasunami H, Morio K, Hamada N, Nishioka A, Ogawa Y: Role of diffusion-weighted imaging in evaluating therapeutic efficacy after transcatheter arterial chemoembolization for hepatocellular carcinoma. Oncol Rep 2010;24:727–732.
58 De Santis M, Alborino S, Tartoni PL, Torricelli P, Casolo A, Romagnoli R: Effects of lipiodol retention on MRI signal intensity from hepatocellular carcinoma and surrounding liver treated by chemoembolization. Eur Radiol 1997;7:10–16.
59 Nasu K, Kuroki Y, Nawano S, Kuroki S, Tsukamoto T, Yamamoto S, Motoori K, Ueda T: Hepatic metastases: diffusion-weighted sensitivity-encoding versus SPIO-enhanced MR imaging. Radiology 2006;239:122–130.

Oncology

Oncology 2013;84(suppl 1):64–68
DOI: 10.1159/000345892

Published online: February 20, 2013

Biomarker Studies on Radiotherapy to Hepatocellular Carcinoma

Chiao-Ling Tsai[a] Albert C. Koong[c] Feng-Ming Hsu[a] Madeline Graber[c]
I-Sin Chen[a] Jason Chia-Hsien Cheng[a, b]

[a]Division of Radiation Oncology, Department of Oncology, National Taiwan University Hospital, and
[b]Graduate Institute of Oncology, National Taiwan University College of Medicine, Taipei, Taiwan, ROC;
[c]Department of Radiation Oncology, Stanford University School of Medicine, Stanford University, Stanford, Calif., USA

Key Words
Hepatocellular carcinoma · Radiotherapy · Biomarker · Proximity ligation assay

Abstract
Radiotherapy (RT) has been gradually integrated into the multimodality treatment for hepatocellular carcinoma (HCC). The various patterns of failure in HCC patients undergoing RT drive the need of effective biomarkers to guide treatment decisions. Limited numbers of biomarkers have been investigated in HCC, with even fewer of them for patients treated by RT. Serum or plasma biomarkers measured by enzyme-linked immunosorbent assay were the most common practice. Of particular interest are those biomarkers that are detectable early in the course of radiotherapy which correlated with ultimate clinical outcome. Functional magnetic resonance imaging (MRI) is increasingly used to evaluate the imaging pattern indicative of disease control following RT. Positron emission tomography shows that pre-RT standard uptake values associate with various types of recurrence after treatment. Proximity ligation assay (PLA) is evolving with the unique features of dual-probe identification, ligation and amplification to allow the small volume of serum/plasma samples for evaluating multiple biomarkers. We demonstrate the screening work of biomarkers by PLA with pre- and post-RT serum samples from HCC patients undergoing RT. Efforts are being made to search for the potential biomarkers for HCC patients treated by RT.

Introduction

Molecular biological markers for treatment response demonstrate great potential for monitoring the therapeutic effect, and even for predicting outcome early in the treatment course. For hepatocellular carcinoma (HCC), one of the most common and intractable malignancies worldwide, useful biomarkers to predict treatment response are needed, especially for radiotherapy (RT). RT plays an increasingly important role in the multimodality management of HCC patients, and appropriate patient selection is critical to optimize the use of RT [1–6]. Traditionally, α-fetoprotein has been widely accepted as a surrogate for disease status. Unfortunately, serum α-fetoprotein level is far from a perfect predictive marker [7]. Because of technological advances in high-throughput screening, new insights into pathological, genetic and molecular events in this disease have become evident. Imaging technological improvements have also provided functional dynamic contrast-enhanced (DCE) and diffusion-weighted (DW) magnetic resonance imaging (MRI) and positron emission tomography (PET) as new techniques for assessing the tumor response [8]. Proximity ligation assay (PLA) is an evolving technique with its unique features of sensitive dual-probe identification, multiplex platform and minimal required sample volume for testing multiple biomarkers [9]. This review summarizes recent studies on biomarkers of RT to HCC to help understand their roles in choosing the most appropriate therapy.

KARGER
Fax +41 61 306 12 34
E-Mail karger@karger.com
www.karger.com

0030–2414/13/0847–0064$38.00/0

Accessible online at:
www.karger.com/ocl

Jason Chia-Hsien Cheng, MD, PhD
Division of Radiation Oncology, Department of Oncology
National Taiwan University Hospital
No. 7 Chung-Shan South Road, Taipei 10002, Taiwan (ROC)
E-Mail jasoncheng@ntu.edu.tw

Serum Biomarkers for HCC

The composition of the serum proteome of cancer patients changes with radiation treatment. In a study by Menard et al. [10], serum was collected before and during a course of radiation therapy from 68 cancer patients. High-resolution surface-enhanced laser desorption and ionization-time of flight (SELDI-TOF) mass spectrometry was used to generate proteomic profiles of unfractionated serum samples using an immobilized metal ion-affinity chromatography nickel-affinity chip surface. Using direct identification techniques of albumin-bound peptides, known as SELDI-TOF finger-prints, 23 protein fragments/peptides were uniquely detected in the radiation exposure group, including an interleukin (IL)-6 precursor protein. Similarly, in the in vivo cirrhotic rat model, the increase of heparanase precursor and the decrease of hepatocyte growth factor (HGF) were commonly shown in liver tissue and serum following irradiation [11].

In a series of serum samples from 37 hepatitis C viral carrier patients before developing HCC, with HCC and following radiofrequency ablation of the tumor, 13 SELDI peaks changed significantly during HCC development [12]. β_2-Microglobulin, a protein previously reported to be markedly elevated in patients with virus-related HCC, was also the most significant HCC-associated proteomic feature in this study. With regards to tumor progression, serum connective tissue growth factor (CTGF), lens culinaris agglutinin A-reactive fraction of AFP, and des-gamma carboxy prothrombin were proposed to reflect different features of the progression in patients with HCC [13, 14].

Sorafenib, an orally active multikinase inhibitor, was the first agent demonstrated to have efficacy in improving the survival of patients with advanced HCC. It inhibits the signaling pathways related to proliferation and proangiogenesis. Miyahara et al. [15] demonstrated that higher baseline angiopoietin-2, follistatin, granulocyte colony-stimulating factor, HGF, leptin, platelet-derived growth factor-BB, platelet endothelial cell adhesion molecule-1 and vascular endothelial growth factor (VEGF) correlated with progression of disease in HCC patients treated with sorafenib. Higher levels of cytokines correlated with worse treatment response. Progression-free survival (PFS) was significantly shorter in patients with high levels of angiopoietin-2, G-CFS, HGF and leptin.

Few studies have identified the significance of serum biomarkers for HCC patients undergoing RT. Given the different patterns of failure in these patients, including the irradiated tumor response, intrahepatic recurrence and extrahepatic metastases [16, 17], effective biomarkers to guide subsequent treatment decisions are critical. Biomarkers should reflect the underlying biology of the irradiated microenvironment, such as sublethal damage of irradiated tumor [18] or bystander effect of radiation-induced cytokines on hepatitis viral reactivation [19–21]. In a phase II study, the serum cytokines from advanced HCC patients treated with concurrent RT and thalidomide were compared with those with RT alone [22]. Among all prognostic factors, only the baseline IL-6 and stem cell-derived factor-1 (SDF-1) levels at week 2 were independent factors associated with the PFS of HCC patients undergoing RT. Stem cell-derived factor-1 level <90% of the baseline level at 1 month after RT was significantly associated with better overall survival (OS).

Functional MRI

Functional DCE-MRI and DW-MRI have been introduced as a new imaging modality to assess tumor response after embolization in HCC patients. With pathologic verification of the degree of tumor necrosis, DW-MRI can quantify tumor necrosis by generating apparent diffusion coefficient maps after chemoembolization. The functional capability of DW-MRI appears to be superior to gadolinium-enhanced MRI [23]. Chung et al. [11] used functional MRI to measure changes in tumor activity at the time of treatment, and compared them to tumor structural changes on conventional MRI after 1- and 3-month follow-up periods. Patients whose intratumoral apparent diffusion coefficient values increased or decreased by >15% were more likely to have a favorable anatomical tumor response.

Liang et al. [24] evaluated 19 patients with advanced HCC undergoing RT. All patients received a DCE, turbo fast low-angle shot MR sequence before RT, at 2 weeks of RT and 1 month later. Initial first-pass enhancement slopes and peak enhancement ratios were measured. In the parenchyma, an increased slope at week 2 was associated with intrahepatic recurrence outside the radiation fields or with progression at distant sites. The signal intensities of contrast enhancement in the hepatic parenchyma at week 2 of RT were associated with local tumor responses.

Positron Emission Tomography

Cancer imaging by PET using fluorine-18-fluoro-2-deoxyglucose (FDG) is based on the observation that most cancers metabolize glucose at an abnormally high rate [25]. Increasing evidence suggests that quantification of changes in FDG uptake may provide an early and sensitive pharmacodynamic marker of the tumoricidal effect of antiproliferative anticancer drugs [26]. In HCC, FDG uptake evaluated by pretreatment PET was associated with tumor differentiation, recurrences and survival after resection, transplantation or chemoembolization [27–29]. FDG-PET was also used for predicting the outcome of sorafenib treatment [30]. A total of 62 patients receiving sorafenib monotherapy for advanced HCC underwent FDG-PET/CT scanning before treatment. The low standard uptake value (SUV) group, defined as maximum SUV (SUV_{max}) <5.0, showed significantly better OS and PFS.

Rapidly proliferating tumors tend to have more aggressive biological behavior and are also more radiosensitive. These characteristics may have translated into a favorable response to RT in the high-SUV ratio group [31]. The SUVs of FDG-PET were obtained from tumor and normal liver tissues for calculating the ratios of SUV_{Tumor}/SUV_{Liver} in 35 HCC patients before RT. Patients with an initially higher SUV ratio (≥2.5) resulted in better response rates than those with a lower SUV ratio. However, the impact of higher SUV ratios did not translate into improved survival, because intrahepatic and distant metastases likely affected the survival. The SUV ratios on pre-RT FDG-PET may help identify HCC patients who are likely to respond to RT.

When combining chemotherapy with RT, tumor SUV_{max} had a good correlation with prognosis [32]. Kim et al. [32] analyzed pretreatment tumor SUV_{max} from 107 locally advanced HCC patients treated with concurrent chemoradiotherapy. Patients with lower tumor SUV_{max} (<6.1) had a higher disease control rate, PFS and OS than those with higher SUV_{max}.

Proximity Ligation Assay

PLA has been developed as a multiplexed protein detection method in which multiple proteins may be detected via unique nucleic-acid identifiers and subsequently quantified by quantitative real-time polymerase chain reaction (qPCR) [9]. The liquid-phase technique uses a pair of proximity probes each composed of an antibody linked to an oligonucleotide. Such a pair allows the hybridization of one connecting oligonucleotide to both probes. It enables the enzymatic ligation of both probes and forms the target reported amplicon for qPCR. PLA has several advantages as compared to other solid-phase methods. Because of the dual-probe nucleic acid assay, PLA has negligible antibody cross-reactivity signal. Multiplex PLA is superior to the existing bead-based platforms for its scalability, with theoretically no upper limit to multiplexing. PLA requires only a few microliters of the sample to test multiple biomarkers. Before the verification of absolute concentration for the specific biomarkers, PLA may be a good screening tool by using the insignificant proportion of samples.

PLA for Cancer Patients

Efforts have been made by use of multiplex PLA to search for the potential serum or plasma biomarkers for various cancers. With the limited volumes of blood samples from cancer patients, it is rarely possible to screen for biomarkers by enzyme-linked immunosorbent assay (ELISA) requiring substantial sample volumes. Multiplex PLA is capable of assaying several biomarkers with only a few microliters of plasma/serum. Such a unique requirement for PLA makes it advantageous to screen the biomarkers for cancer patients. With the selected biomarkers showing their significance in the screening phase by PLA, the subsequent verification by ELISA for the absolute concentration is essential.

Most studies on serum/plasma PLA of cancer patients were from the selected patients to support the proposed methodology, while few studies actually used PLA as a screening tool for biomarkers to differentiate cancer patients from healthy controls. The Stanford group was one of the first groups to develop and apply PLA in a biomarker discovery effort for cancer patients. Fredriksson et al. [33] used 4 multiplex panels with each for detecting 6 or 7 markers, to compare 18 pancreatic cancer patients with 19 matched healthy controls and 20 ovarian cancer patients with 20 matched healthy controls. CA19-9 and CA125 were the most significant biomarkers to differentiate patients from controls for the two cancers, respectively. Concordant results were found in the literature for most of the markers tested by PLA. Chang et al. [34] tested the plasma levels of 21 biomarkers in 52 locally advanced pancreatic cancer patients and 43 age-matched controls by multiplex PLA. A three-biomarker panel (CA19-9, osteopontin and chitinase 3-like 1) was more predictive of pancreatic cancer than CA19-9 alone in locally advanced disease. Furthermore, the CEA/CA125 panel significantly predicted survival. To date, however, there have not been any studies comparing various biomarkers by PLA in patients before and after cancer therapy.

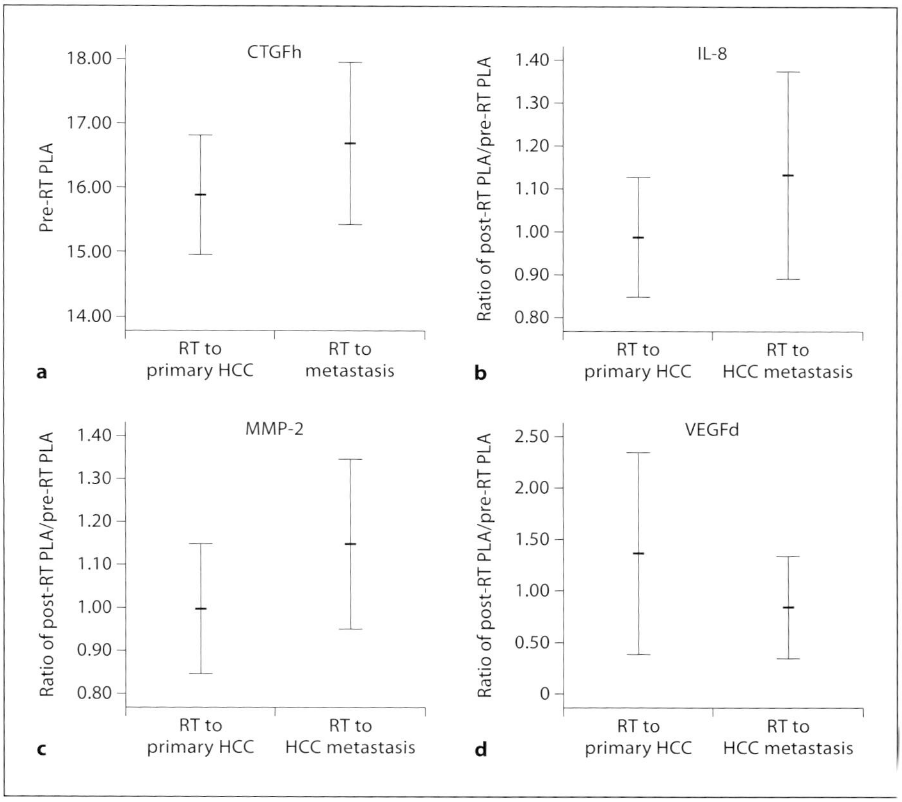

Fig. 1. Serum levels of 4 biomarkers with statistical significance between HCC patients undergoing RT to the primary liver tumor and RT to the extrahepatic metastasis. The data are presented with mean ± standard deviation of $\log_2$ PLA units. Significantly higher pre-RT serum level of CTGF in RT to metastasis than RT to primary HCC, $p = 0.019$ (**a**); significantly lower post-RT/pre-RT ratios of IL-8, $p = 0.039$ (**b**) and MMP-2, $p = 0.008$ (**c**) as well as higher VEGFd, $p = 0.053$ (**d**) in RT to primary HCC than RT to metastasis.

Preliminary Effort in PLA of HCC Patients Undergoing RT

With our prospectively collected pre-RT and post-RT serum samples from 45 HCC patients undergoing RT, we used multiplex PLA 8-marker panels to screen a total of 51 biomarkers. Twenty-nine patients had RT to the intrahepatic tumor, while 16 patients had RT to the extrahepatic metastasis. Each patient had serum samples collected pre-RT and within 1 month post-RT. Among the tested markers, CTGF showed a significant difference in pre-RT serum levels between the two groups. Patients with RT to intrahepatic HCC had higher $\log_2$ PLA units than those with RT to extrahepatic metastasis (fig. 1a). The changes in $\log_2$ PLA units of the screened biomarkers between pre- and post-RT serum samples were shown with the ratios of post-RT/pre-RT $\log_2$ units. Patients with RT to primary HCC had significantly lower ratios of IL-8 (fig. 1b) and MMP-2 (fig. 1c) and a higher ratio of VEGFd (fig. 1d) than those with RT to metastasis. These findings implied the association of certain biomarkers with extrahepatic metastasis, and the angiogenesis-related mechanism of metastasis from HCC. These results need to be confirmed by other methods of detection such as ELISA.

Conclusion

The potential biomarkers guiding the patterns of failure of HCC patients undergoing RT are not widely available. Serum/plasma markers, functional MRI and FDG-PET have been selectively used to predict disease outcome. Multiplex PLA may have the advantage of screening multiple biomarkers with limited sample volume. More studies are needed to validate and determine the significance of these biomarkers before they become routinely used for clinical decision making in HCC patients.

Disclosure Statement

The authors declare no conflict of interest.

References

1 Cha J, Seong J: Radiotherapeutic strategies according to the BCLC stages in hepatocellular carcinoma. Liver Cancer, in press.

2 Bae SH, Kim MS, Cho CK, Kim KB, Lee DH, Han CJ, et al: Feasibility and efficacy of stereotactic ablative radiotherapy for Barcelona clinical liver cancer-C hepatocellular carcinoma. Liver Cancer 2012;1:112.

3 Jiang GL: Hepatic proliferation after irradiation injuries. Liver Cancer 2012;1:120.

4 Park JH, Yoon SM, Lim YS, Kim SY, Shim JH, Kim KM, et al: A two-week schedule of hypofractionated radiotherapy in patients with small hepatocellular carcinoma: efficacy and clinical outcomes. Liver Cancer 2012;1:131.

5 Yoon HI, Lee IJ, Pyun HO, Han KH, Seong J: Matched pair analysis comparing the clinical outcome of hypofractionated radiotherapy with tomotherapy and 3-dimensional conventional radiotherapy in locally advanced hepatocellular carcinoma. Liver Cancer 2012;1:137.

6 Yu JI, Park HC, Yoon SM, Kim TH, Seong J, Jang HS, et al: Multicenter validation study of the prognostic index for portal vein tumor thrombosis in patients with hepatocellular carcinoma treated with radiation therapy: comparison among the Okuda, CLIP, CUPI and JIS staging systems (KROG 11-05). Liver Cancer 2012;1:138.

7 Farinati F, Marino D, De Giorgio M, Baldan A, Cantarini M, Cursaro C, et al: Diagnostic and prognostic role of alpha-fetoprotein in hepatocellular carcinoma: both or neither? Am J Gastroenterol 2006;101:524–532.

8 Kamel IR, Bluemke DA, Eng J, Liapi E, Messersmith W, Reyes DK, et al: The role of functional MR imaging in the assessment of tumor response after chemoembolization in patients with hepatocellular carcinoma. J Vasc Interv Radiol 2006;17:505–512.

9 Fredriksson S, Dixon W, Ji H, Koong AC, Mindrinos M, Davis RW: Multiplexed protein detection by proximity ligation for cancer biomarker validation. Nat Methods 2007;4:327–329.

10 Menard C, Johann D, Lowenthal M, Muanza T, Sproull M, Ross S, et al: Discovering clinical biomarkers of ionizing radiation exposure with serum proteomic analysis. Cancer Res 2006;66:1844–1850.

11 Chung SI, Seong J, Park YN, Kim WW, Oh HJ, Han KH: Identification of proteins indicating radiation-induced hepatic toxicity in cirrhotic rats. J Radiat Res 2010;51:643–650.

12 Ward DG, Cheng Y, N'Kontchou G, Thar TT, Barget N, Wei W, et al: Preclinical and post-treatment changes in the HCC-associated serum proteome. Br J Cancer 2006;95:1379–1383.

13 Toyoda H, Kumada T, Osaki Y, Oka H, Urano F, Kudo M, et al: Staging hepatocellular carcinoma by a novel scoring system (BALAD score) based on serum markers. Clin Gastroenterol Hepatol 2006;4:1528–1536.

14 Wang GB, Zhou XY, Yuan T, Xie J, Guo LP, Gao N, et al: Significance of serum connective tissue growth factor in patients with hepatocellular carcinoma and relationship with angiogenesis. World J Surg 2010;34:2411–2417.

15 Miyahara K, Nouso K, Tomoda T, Kobayashi S, Hagihara H, Kuwaki K, et al: Predicting the treatment effect of sorafenib using serum angiogenesis markers in patients with hepatocellular carcinoma. J Gastroenterol Hepatol 2011;26:1604–1611.

16 Cheng JC, Chuang VP, Cheng SH, Huang AT, Lin YM, Cheng TI, et al: Local radiotherapy with or without transcatheter arterial chemoembolization for patients with unresectable hepatocellular carcinoma. Int J Radiat Oncol Biol Phys 2000;47:435–442.

17 Lee IJ, Seong J: Radiotherapeutic strategies in the management of hepatocellular carcinoma. Oncology 2011;81(suppl 1):123–133.

18 Chou CH, Teng CM, Tzen KY, Chang YC, Chen JH, Cheng JC: MMP-9 from sublethally irradiated tumor promotes Lewis lung carcinoma cell invasiveness and pulmonary metastasis. Oncogene 2012;31:458–468.

19 Cheng JC, Wu JK, Lee PC, Liu HS, Jian JJ, Lin YM, et al: Biologic susceptibility of hepatocellular carcinoma patients treated with radiotherapy to radiation-induced liver disease. Int J Radiat Oncol Biol Phys 2004;60:1502–1509.

20 Chou CH, Chen PJ, Lee PH, Cheng AL, Hsu HC, Cheng JC: Radiation-induced hepatitis B virus reactivation in liver mediated by the bystander effect from irradiated endothelial cells. Clin Cancer Res 2007;13:851–857.

21 Dupret JM, Grant DM: Site-directed mutagenesis of recombinant human arylamine N-acetyltransferase expressed in *Escherichia coli*. Evidence for direct involvement of Cys68 in the catalytic mechanism of polymorphic human NAT2. J Biol Chem 1992;267:7381–7385.

22 Ch'ang HJ, Hsu C, Chen CH, Chang YH, Chang JS, Chen LT: Phase II study of concomitant thalidomide during radiotherapy for hepatocellular carcinoma. Int J Radiat Oncol Biol Phys 2012;82:817–825.

23 Kamel IR, Bluemke DA, Ramsey D, Abusedera M, Torbenson M, Eng J, et al: Role of diffusion-weighted imaging in estimating tumor necrosis after chemoembolization of hepatocellular carcinoma. Am J Roentgenol 2003;181:708–710.

24 Liang PC, Ch'ang HJ, Hsu C, Tseng SS, Shih TT, Wu Liu T: Dynamic MRI signals in the second week of radiotherapy relate to treatment outcomes of hepatocellular carcinoma: a preliminary result. Liver Int 2007;27:516–528.

25 Rigo P, Paulus P, Kaschten BJ, Hustinx R, Bury T, Jerusalem G, et al: Oncological applications of positron emission tomography with fluorine-18 fluorodeoxyglucose. Eur J Nuclear Med 1996;23:1641–1674.

26 Young H, Baum R, Cremerius U, Herholz K, Hoekstra O, Lammertsma AA, et al: Measurement of clinical and subclinical tumour response using [^{18}F]-fluorodeoxyglucose and positron emission tomography: review and 1999 EORTC recommendations. Eur J Cancer 1999;35:1773–1782.

27 Seo S, Hatano E, Higashi T, Hara T, Tada M, Tamaki N, et al: Fluorine-18 fluorodeoxyglucose positron emission tomography predicts tumor differentiation, P-glycoprotein expression, and outcome after resection in hepatocellular carcinoma. Clin Cancer Res 2007;13(2 Pt 1):427–433.

28 Lee SD, Kim SH, Kim YK, Kim C, Kim SK, Han SS, et al: ^{18}F-FDG-PET/CT predicts early tumor recurrence in living donor liver transplantation for hepatocellular carcinoma. Transpl Int 2012, E-pub ahead of print.

29 Kim HO, Kim JS, Shin YM, Ryu JS, Lee YS, Lee SG: Evaluation of metabolic characteristics and viability of lipiodolized hepatocellular carcinomas using ^{18}F-FDG PET/CT. J Nuclear Med 2010;51:1849–1856.

30 Lee JH, Park JY, Kim do Y, Ahn SH, Han KH, Seo HJ, et al: Prognostic value of ^{18}F-FDG PET for hepatocellular carcinoma patients treated with sorafenib. Liver Int 2011;31:1144–1149.

31 Kim JW, Seong J, Yun M, Lee IJ, Yoon HI, Cho HJ, et al: Usefulness of positron emission tomography with fluorine-18-fluorodeoxyglucose in predicting treatment response in unresectable hepatocellular carcinoma patients treated with external beam radiotherapy. Int J Radiat Oncol Biol Phys 2012;82:1172–1178.

32 Kim BK, Kang WJ, Kim JK, Seong J, Park JY, Kim do Y, et al: ^{18}F-fluorodeoxyglucose uptake on positron emission tomography as a prognostic predictor in locally advanced hepatocellular carcinoma. Cancer 2011;117:4779–4787.

33 Fredriksson S, Horecka J, Brustugun OT, Schlingemann J, Koong AC, Tibshirani R, et al: Multiplexed proximity ligation assays to profile putative plasma biomarkers relevant to pancreatic and ovarian cancer. Clin Chem 2008;54:582–589.

34 Chang ST, Zahn JM, Horecka J, Kunz PL, Ford JM, Fisher GA, et al: Identification of a biomarker panel using a multiplex proximity ligation assay improves accuracy of pancreatic cancer diagnosis. J Transl Med 2009;7:105.

Oncology

Oncology 2013;84(suppl 1):69–74
DOI: 10.1159/000345893

Published online: February 20, 2013

Is It Time to Adopt External Beam Radiotherapy in the NCCN Guidelines as a Therapeutic Strategy for Intermediate/Advanced Hepatocellular Carcinoma?

Wei Jiang Zhao-Chong Zeng

Department of Radiation Oncology, Zhongshan Hospital, Fudan University, Shanghai, PR China

Key Words
Radiation therapy · Hepatocellular carcinoma · Guidelines

Abstract

Objective: External beam radiotherapy (EBRT) is recommended as a therapeutic strategy for stage III hepatocellular carcinoma (HCC) in national guidelines of the Chinese Society of Liver Disease and in Korea Liver Cancer Study Group practice guidelines, but has not been considered a therapeutic option for HCC in Western countries. In this study, we review evidence supporting EBRT as an option for HCC treatment. ***Methods:*** Retrospective investigation was made of 775 patient records of intermediate/advanced HCC treated in our hospital during the last 10 years, including 98 patients with confined intrahepatic tumor, 181 with portal vein (PV) or inferior vena cava (IVC) tumor thrombi, 191 with lymph node metastases, 55 with adrenal gland metastases, 205 with bone metastases, 13 with lung metastases and 32 with brain metastases. ***Results:*** Transcatheter arterial chemoembolization combined with radiotherapy was found to constitute an improved therapeutic strategy for unresectable but confined intrahepatic HCC with poor lipid accumulation. Survival of HCC patients with PV/IVC tumor thrombi was prolonged to 10.7 months by radiotherapy, and it was 8.0 months in patients with abdominal lymph node metastasis. Radiotherapy also shrinks adrenal and lung metastatic HCC lesions, resulting in median survival times of 13.6 and progression-free survival of 13.4 months, respectively. In bone metastatic HCC, radiotherapy significantly relieved symptoms, although median survival time was only 7.4 months. Radiotherapy is effective for treatment of intermediate/advanced stages of HCC. Although our finding is based only on retrospective analysis, no therapeutic option that provides better treatment than EBRT in this indication has thus far been identified. Because sorafenib has been recommended as a treatment strategy by the National Comprehensive Cancer Network (NCCN) for HCC, we compared the survival after EBRT with sorafenib treatment on the basis of published clinical data. From this comparison, we found that EBRT treatment was more effective than sorafenib for improving patient survival when tested on tumors of comparable metastatic size. ***Conclusion:*** Based on the evidence reviewed, we propose that EBRT be included in the NCCN guideline as a treatment strategy for intermediate/advanced HCC.

Introduction

Hepatocellular carcinoma (HCC) is a highly prevalent and lethal neoplasia. The management of HCC has significantly improved over the last few years. Patients with early HCC have excellent chances for curative cancer treatment. However, most cases of the disease are detected at an intermediate to advanced stage. With recent de-

KARGER

Fax +41 61 306 12 34
E-Mail karger@karger.com
www.karger.com

0030–2414/13/0847–0069$38.00/0

Accessible online at:
www.karger.com/ocl

Zhao-Chong Zeng, MD
Zhongshan Hospital, Fudan University
136 Yi Xue Yuan Road
Shanghai 200032 (PR China)
E-Mail zeng.zhaochong@zs-hospital.sh.cn

velopments in radiotherapy [1–6] technology involving precise delivery of focused high-doses on partial volume of the liver, or sparing organs at risk, we ask what is the role of radiotherapy in the treatment strategy of HCC? In this review, we shall discuss mainly clinical results with which we have had direct experience in practice at our hospital.

Benefit of EBRT in Early-Stage HCC Has Not Been Defined

Current options for the treatment of early HCC conforming to authoritative guidelines, such as the Milan criteria and Barcelona Clinic Liver Cancer (BCLC) staging system, apply to liver transplantation, surgical resection, transcatheter arterial chemoembolization (TACE) and percutaneous tumor ablation [7, 8]. Five-year survival rates can be achieved in 50–80% of cases by these treatments [7]. Stereotactic body radiation therapy (SBRT) has emerged as a promising noninvasive therapy. A limited number of clinical trials examining the use of SBRT in patients with HCC have been reported and the 3-year survival rates can reach approximately 60% [9, 10]. However, those data are limited by the small number and unresectable patients. The application of EBRT in early HCC needs to be further investigated.

EBRT Is Recommended as a Therapeutic Strategy for Stage III HCC

According to the BCLC Staging and Treatment Strategy, patients at intermediate and advanced stages account for approximately 50% of all HCC cases [11], and in approximately a further 15% of patients, extrahepatic metastases is detected in the follow-up period after the initial diagnosis of intrahepatic HCC [12]. In the 2011 Chinese Guidelines for diagnosis and treatment of HCC it is recommended that EBRT should be a treatment strategy for intermediate/advanced HCC [13] and the 2009 Korean Liver Cancer Study Group practice guidelines [14]. This is supported by a series of reports on radiotherapy in HCC. Using the search terms 'hepatocellular carcinoma' and 'radiotherapy', we retrieved 902 related articles in PubMed dated until 2011. We then performed retrospective investigations of 775 patients with intermediate/advanced HCC treated in our hospital in the last 10 years, including 98 patients with confined intrahepatic tumor, 181 with portal vein (PV) or inferior vena cava (IVC) tumor thrombi, 191 with lymph node metastases, 55 with adrenal gland metastases, 205 with bone metastases, 13 with lung metastases and 32 with brain metastases. Although higher evidence-based medicine is lacking, no therapeutic option that provides better treatment than EBRT in this indication has thus far been identified. Therefore, palliative radiotherapy may be a potential remedy for these patients.

Radiotherapy May Be a Complement in Patients of Poor Lipiodol Accumulation after TACE for Unresectable but Confined Intrahepatic HCC

TACE does not induce complete or massive necrosis of HCC tumors greater than 5 cm in diameter. Accordingly, following treatment with TACE, patients with large tumors have significantly worse survival rates than those with smaller tumors. Because larger tumors have both arterial and portal blood supply that allows tumor cells to remain viable even following complete arterial embolization by TACE, these cells become the source of recurrence and metastasis after treatment. But the combination with EBRT holds promise for overcoming this challenge. Our retrospective study suggests that the median overall survival (OS) of patients treated with radiotherapy was 23.1 months, significantly better than the nonradiotherapy group [15, 16]. Similar findings have been reported by other investigators, with a 2-year survival rate of 50–60% [17, 18].

Radiotherapy Can Improve Survival in HCC Patients with PV/IVC Tumor Thrombus

HCC patients with PV tumor thrombus have a poor prognosis with median survival time of only 2.4–2.7 months without treatment. Our latest retrospective data show that the median survival of 181 patients with PV and/or IVC tumor thrombi who were referred for EBRT was 10.7 months [19]. A study employing a nonradiotherapy group at our clinic during the same period shows the median survival and the 1-year survival rates were 8.9 months and 34.4% in the EBRT group, and 4 months and 11.4% in the non-EBRT group, respectively [20, 21]. Data from 281 HCC patients with PVT treated by radiotherapy in Korea have shown a median OS of 11.6 months [22].

Radiotherapy Decreases the Mortality of HCC Patients with Abdominal Lymph Node Metastasis

Most patients with lymph node metastasis of HCC are no longer eligible for surgical resection, TACE, percutaneous ethanol injection or radiofrequency ablation. We studied HCC patients with abdominal lymph node me-

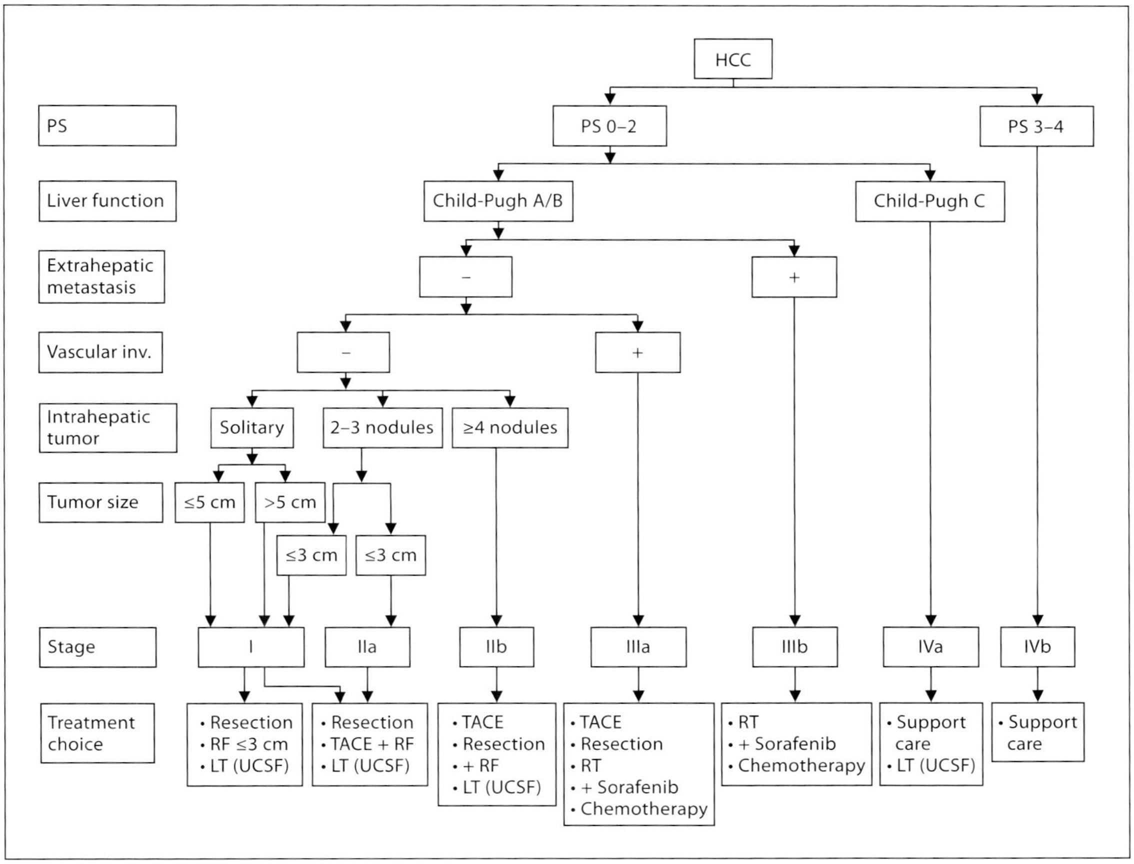

Fig. 1. Strategy for staging and treatment assignment in patients diagnosed with HCC according to the proposal from the Chinese Society of Liver Disease. PS = Performance status

tastasis either treated or not treated by EBRT in the same period. The effect on survival outcome was significant, and EBRT can reduce mortality resulting from nodal involvement [23]. Our latest data of 191 such patients shows that EBRT provides a median OS of 8.0 months [24]. A similar result was confirmed by a report from Korea [25].

Radiotherapy Shrinks Adrenal Metastatic HCC Lesions

The most effective treatment modality for adrenal metastasis of HCC remains unclear. Based on case reports, previous approaches attempted for the management of this condition include surgical resection, TACE and percutaneous ethanol injection. Surgical resection is usually not considered upon diagnosis of adrenal metastasis due to the presence of unresectable intrahepatic tumors, tumor thrombi, lymph node involvement and/or synchronous distant metastases to bone or lung. Theoretically, TACE should be effective in treating adrenal metastases because metastatic lesions are hypervascular, similar to primary HCC. However, TACE is not performed in this case because catheterization of the adrenal arteries and complete embolization of the adrenal gland presents anatomical and technical challenges. In our records, there were 55 patients with adrenal gland metastases from HCC who were treated by radiotherapy, and the median survival time was 13.6 months [26, 27].

Radiotherapy Significantly Improves Quality of Life of Patients with Bone Metastases from HCC

Of the treatment choices for bone metastases from HCC, including surgery, internal and external radiation therapy, bisphosphonates and analgesic drugs, it remains unclear which is optimal. In practice, radiotherapy has been generally accepted as effective in palliating painful bone metastases and is less costly. Here, alleviation of

Table 1. Comparison of median survival benefits (months) between sorafenib and radiotherapy for intermediate/advanced HCC

	Asia-Pacific trial		SHARP		EBRT	
	sorafenib	placebo	sorafenib	placebo	China	Korea
Plus TACE for intrahepatic tumor	29.7 [36] (Ø ≤7 cm)	>29.7 [36]	–	–	23.1 [15] (max. Ø 5–20 cm)	32 [37] (max. Ø 5–7 cm)
Median OS						
PV tumor thrombus	5.6 [34]	4.1 [34]	10.7 [35]	7.9 [35]	9.7 [21]	11.6 [22]
Lung metastasis	5.6 [34]	4.2 [34]	10.7 [35]	7.9 [35]	16.7[1] [30]	12.3 [31]
Lymph node metastasis	5.6 [34]	3.2 [34]	10.7 [35]	7.9 [35]	8.0 [24]	10 [25]

Values represent survival in months. Publications in the reference list are cited in square brackets. Ø = Diameter.
[1] Mean survival.

symptoms is the purpose of radiotherapy. Pain relief was reported in 99.5% of HCC patients with bone metastases in our cohort, and the median survival was 7.4 months [28]; however, there was no evidence that EBRT prolongs survival in these patients.

EBRT Appears to Be a Viable Treatment Choice for Pulmonary Metastases

The lung is the most common organ affected by extrahepatic metastases from HCC. Metastatic lesions in the lung commonly tend to be multiple, but progress more slowly than primary intrahepatic lesions. Thus, death from lung metastases occurs in no more than 20% of HCC patients [29]. In our cohort, there were 13 HCC patients with pulmonary metastases treated by three-dimensional conformal radiotherapy from a traditional accelerator, and we observed a 2-year survival rate of 70% [30]. Helical tomotherapy has been developed to more easily achieve radiotherapy for multiple pulmonary metastases. A Korean group reported tomotherapy for metastatic lesions in HCC patients using a dose of 51.03 Gy (range 30–57.61) in 10 fractions. A complete response rate of 26.3% of pulmonary lesions was observed and the median OS was 12.3 months [31].

EBRT Is the Major Palliative Treatment in the Management of Brain Metastases

Brain metastasis of HCC is frequently associated with hemorrhage (so-called 'tumor stroke'), because HCC itself is hypervascular and most patients have coagulopathy due to liver cirrhosis. Patients must undergo radiotherapy immediately upon diagnosis of brain metastasis. A median survival time of 4.5 months has been reported, and 1-year survival was 15.6% in 32 patients with brain metastases from HCC who received EBRT [32]. A Korean study reported that the median survival of patients with brain metastasis was 6.8 weeks [33]. Classified according to treatment modality, median survival was 33.6 weeks for patients who underwent resection and received EBRT; 10.0 weeks for patients who received surgery, gamma-knife surgery or EBRT only, and 2.0 weeks for those who received only steroids, and there were significant differences.

Comparison between Sorafenib and Radiotherapy for Intermediate/Advanced HCC

Sorafenib has been recommended as a treatment strategy by the National Comprehensive Cancer Network (NCCN) for HCC. We reviewed the representative studies on sorafenib both in Asian and Western countries. In the phase III Sorafenib Asia-Pacific trial of 226 patients with advanced HCC, median OS was 5.6 months in patients with macrovascular invasion and/or extrahepatic spread who received sorafenib [34]. In the Sorafenib HCC Assessment Randomized Protocol (SHARP) trial in advanced HCC, median OS was 10.7 months in the sorafenib group and 7.9 months with placebo [35]. Our comparative analysis of treatment of advanced HCC with sorafenib versus EBRT, using data from our practice and that published from Korea, is summarized in table 1 [15, 21, 22, 24, 25, 30, 31, 36, 37]. We can see that besides the better local control achieved by EBRT in HCC, which is a known effect, EBRT may provide an advantage over sorafenib on survival in some types of HCC.

Besides efficacy, EBRT has a significant economic advantage over sorafenib. A deterministic incremental cost-effectiveness ratio of 64,754 GBP per quality-adjusted life-year was generated in the base case for sorafenib in an economic analysis based on licensed indication submitted by the manufacturer [38]. Therefore, the high cost and modest efficacy of sorafenib prohibits its widespread use. In contrast, EBRT is affordable and recommended as a better therapeutic option.

Perspectives of an Era of Curative Radiotherapy for HCC

With continuing development in the technique of radiotherapy, curative radiotherapy is expected to be available in the future. Use of curative radiotherapy has three criteria: (1) a radical dose is required; (2) no clinical lesions should lie beyond the radiation fields and subclinical volumes should be in the prophylactic range, and (3) the side-effects should be tolerable. Clinicians should consider radical radiotherapy for local HCC in cases where a radical dose can be delivered without severe toxicity. For early HCC, there have been many positive reports of treatment by SBRT for early HCC; however, its value compared to surgery or ablation is not yet well defined.

Reports on radiotherapy for intermediate/advanced HCC mainly focus on palliative treatment. This is because of the difficulty in intermediate/advanced HCC of giving doses over 66 Gy by three-dimensional conformal radiotherapy, which is the mainstream technology. In many cases, such as large tumors or poor liver function, maximum irradiation doses achieved are limited to 40 Gy.

Helical tomotherapy, with advantages of multitarget irradiation and higher precision dose distribution compared to conventional linear accelerators, can deliver any dose distribution required in vivo using spiral computed tomography image guidance. Hence, helical tomotherapy is optimal for unresectable HCC, which usually presents with multiple lesions. The study from Korea on tomotherapy for HCC patients with intra- and extrahepatic lesions (including lung, adrenal gland and soft tissue metastases) reports a median survival of 12.3 months in advanced cases, with an actuarial in-field tumor control rate for 1 year of 79.0%, and no cases of grade 4–5 acute toxicity [31]. We are attempting to deliver radical radiotherapy using tomotherapy simultaneously for PV tumor thrombus and intrahepatic primary lesion in some HCC patients, thus realizing curative radiotherapy in advanced HCC; our investigation is in progress.

Conclusions

Using evidence-based medicine criteria, there is a limited number of high-level studies on EBRT in HCC. However, there is sufficient evidence to suggest that with EBRT we have entered a new era for treatment of intermediate/advanced HCC. Future researches should focus on validation of procedures and improvement in efficacy. We propose that EBRT be considered for inclusion in the NCCN guideline as a treatment strategy for intermediate/advanced HCC.

Disclosure Statement

The authors declare there are no conflicts of interest with respect to any work in this article or its publication.

References

1 Cha J, Seong J: Radiotherapeutic strategies according to the BCLC stages in hepatocellular carcinoma. Liver Cancer 2012;1:216–225.

2 Bae SH, Kim MS, Cho CK, Kim KB, Lee DH, Han CJ, et al: Feasibility and efficacy of stereotactic ablative radiotherapy for Barcelona Clinical Liver Cancer-C hepatocellular carcinoma. Liver Cancer 2012;1:112.

3 Jiang GL: Hepatic proliferation after irradiation injuries. Liver Cancer 2012;1:120.

4 Park JH, Yoon SM, Lim YS, Kim SY, Shim JH, Kim KM, et al: A two-week schedule of hypofractionated radiotherapy in patients with small hepatocellular carcinoma: efficacy and clinical outcomes. Liver Cancer 2012;1:131.

5 Yoon HI, Lee IJ, Pyun HO, Han KH, Seong J: Matched pair analysis comparing the clinical outcome of hypofractionated radiothrapy with tomotherapyand 3-dimensional conventional radiotherapy in locally advanced hepatocellular carcinoma. Liver Cancer 2012;1:137.

6 Yu JI, Park HC, Yoon SM, Kim TH, Seong J, Jang HS, et al: Multicenter validation study of the prognostic index for portal vein tumor thrombosis in patients with hepatocellular carcinoma treated with radiation therapy: comparison among the Okuda, CLIP, CUPI and JIS staging systems (KROG 11-05). Liver Cancer 2012;1:138.

7 de Lope CR, Tremosini S, Forner A, Reig M, Bruix J: Management of HCC. J Hepatol 2012;56(suppl 1):S75–S87.

8 Benson AB 3rd, Abrams TA, Ben-Josef E, Bloomston PM, Botha JF, Clary BM, et al: NCCN clinical practice guidelines in oncology: hepatobiliary cancers. J Natl Compr Cancer Netw 2009;7:350–391.

9 Cardenes HR, Price TR, Perkins SM, Maluccio M, Kwo P, Breen TE, et al: Phase I feasibility trial of stereotactic body radiation therapy for primary hepatocellular carcinoma Clin Transl Oncol 2010;12:218–225.

10 Kwon JH, Bae SH, Kim JY, Choi BO, Jang HS, Jang JW, et al: Long-term effect of stereotactic body radiation therapy for primary hepatocellular carcinoma ineligible for local ablation therapy or surgical resection. Stereotactic radiotherapy for liver cancer. BMC Cancer 2010;10:475.

11 Hsu CY, Hsia CY, Huang YH, Su CW, Lin HC, Lee PC, et al: Selecting an optimal staging system for hepatocellular carcinoma: comparison of 5 currently used prognostic models. Cancer 2010;116:3006–3014.
12 Natsuizaka M, Omura T, Akaike T, Kuwata Y, Yamazaki K, Sato T, et al: Clinical features of hepatocellular carcinoma with extrahepatic metastases. J Gastroenterol Hepatol 2005;20:1781–1787.
13 Ministry of Public Health of the People's Republic of China: Guideline for diagnosis and treatments of hepatocellular carcinoma. Chin Clin Oncol 2011;16:929–946.
14 Korean Liver Cancer Study Group and National Cancer Center, Korea: Practice guidelines for management of hepatocellular carcinoma 2009 (in Korean). Korean J Hepatol 2009;15:391–423.
15 Zeng ZC, Yang P, Wang BL, Sun J, Chen B: Poor lipiodol accumulation is an unfavorable predictor in hepatocellular carcinoma patients treated with combination transcatheter arterial chemoembolization and external beam radiotherapy. Int J Radiat Oncol, Biol, Phys 2011;S2:352–353.
16 Zeng ZC, Tang ZY, Fan J, Zhou J, Qin LX, Ye SL, et al: A comparison of chemoembolization combination with and without radiotherapy for unresectable hepatocellular carcinoma. Cancer J 2004;10:307–316.
17 Mornex F, Girard N, Beziat C, Kubas A, Khodri M, Trepo C, et al: Feasibility and efficacy of high-dose three-dimensional-conformal radiotherapy in cirrhotic patients with small-size hepatocellular carcinoma non-eligible for curative therapies – mature results of the French Phase II RTF-1 trial. Int J Radiat Oncol Biol Phys 2006;66:1152–1158.
18 Mornex F, Girard N, Merle P, Beziat C, Kubas A, Wautot V, et al: Tolerance and efficacy of conformal radiotherapy for hepatocellular carcinoma in cirrhotic patients. Results of the French RTF1 phase II trial (in French). Cancer Radiother 2005;9:470–476.
19 Hou JZ, Zeng ZC, Zhang JY, Fan J, Zhou J, Zeng MS: Influence of tumor thrombus location on the outcome of external-beam radiation therapy in advanced hepatocellular carcinoma with macrovascular invasion. Int J Radiat Oncol Biol Phys 2012;84:362–368.
20 Zeng ZC, Fan J, Tang ZY, Zhou J, Qin LX, Wang JH, et al: A comparison of treatment combinations with and without radiotherapy for hepatocellular carcinoma with portal vein and/or inferior vena cava tumor thrombus. Int J Radiat Oncol Biol Phys 2005;61:432–443.
21 Zeng ZC, Fan J, Tang ZY, Zhou J, Wang JH, Wang BL, et al: Prognostic factors for patients with hepatocellular carcinoma with macroscopic portal vein or inferior vena cava tumor thrombi receiving external-beam radiation therapy. Cancer Sci 2008;99:2510–2517.
22 Yu JI, Park HC, Lim do H, Park W, Yoo BC, Paik SW, et al: Prognostic index for portal vein tumor thrombosis in patients with hepatocellular carcinoma treated with radiation therapy. J Korean Med Sci 2011;26:1014–1022.
23 Zeng ZC, Tang ZY, Fan J, Qin LX, Ye SL, Zhou J, et al: Consideration of role of radiotherapy for lymph node metastases in patients with HCC: retrospective analysis for prognostic factors from 125 patients. Int J Radiat Oncol Biol Phys 2005;63:1067–1076.
24 Chen YX, Zeng ZC, Fan J, Tang ZY, Zhou J, Wang JH, et al: Defining prognositic factors of survival after external beam radiotherapy treatment of hepatocellular carcinoma with lymph node metastases. Clin Transl Oncol DOI: 10.1007/s12094-012-0997-6.
25 Kim K, Chie EK, Kim W, Kim YJ, Yoon JH, Lee HS, et al: Absence of- -smptom and intact liver function are posi-tive prognosticators for patients undergoing radiotherapy for lymph node metastasis from hepatocellular carcinoma. Int J Radiat Oncol Biol Phys 2010;78:729–734.
26 Zeng ZC, Tang ZY, Fan J, Zhou J, Qin LX, Ye SL, et al: Radiation therapy for adrenal gland metastases from hepatocellular carcinoma. Jpn J Clin Oncol 2005;35:61–67.
27 Zhou LY, Zeng ZC, Chen B: Radiotherapy treatment of adrenal gland metastases from hepatocellular carcinoma: clinical features and prognostic factors. BMC Cancer, in press.
28 He J, Zeng ZC, Tang ZY, Fan J, Zhou J, Zeng MS, et al: Clinical features and prognostic factors in patients with bone metastases from hepatocellular carcinoma receiving external beam radiotherapy. Cancer 2009;115: 2710–2720.
29 Kitano K, Murayama T, Sakamoto M, Nagayama K, Ueno K, Murakawa T, Nakajima J: Outcome and survival analysis of pulmonary metastasectomy for hepatocellular carcinoma. Eur J Cardiothorac Surg 2012;41: 376–382.
30 Jiang W, Zeng ZC, Zhang JY, Fan J, Zeng MS, Zhou J: Palliative radiation therapy for pulmonary metastases from hepatocellular carcinoma. Clin Exp Metastasis 2012;29:197–205.
31 Jang JW, Kay CS, You CR, Kim CW, Bae SH, Choi JY, et al: Simultaneous multitarget irradiation using helical tomotherapy for advanced hepatocellular carcinoma with multiple extrahepatic metastases. Int J Radiat Oncol Biol Phys 2009;74:412–418.
32 Qiu SJ, Zeng ZC: Clinical features and prognosis of patients with brain metastasis from hepatocellular carcinoma. Clin Med J China, in press.
33 Choi HJ, Cho BC, Sohn JH, Shin SJ, Kim SH, Kim JH, Yoo NC: Brain metastases from hepatocellular carcinoma: prognostic factors and outcome: brain metastasis from HCC. J Neurooncol 2009;91:307–313.
34 Cheng AL, Guan Z, Chen Z, Tsao CJ, Qin S, Kim JS, et al: Efficacy and safety of sorafenib in patients with advanced hepatocellular carcinoma according to baseline status: subset analyses of the phase III Sorafenib Asia-Pacific trial. Eur J Cancer 2012;48:1452–1465.
35 Llovet JM, Ricci S, Mazzaferro V, Hilgard P, Gane E, Blanc JF, et al: Sorafenib in advanced hepatocellular carcinoma. N Engl J Med 2008;359:378–390.
36 Kudo M, Imanaka K, Chida N, Nakachi K, Tak WY, Takayama T, et al: Phase III study of sorafenib after transarterial chemoembolisation in Japanese and Korean patients with unresectable hepatocellular carcinoma. Eur J Cancer 2011;47:2117–2127.
37 Shim SJ, Seong J, Han KH, Chon CY, Suh CO, Lee JT: Local radiotherapy as a complement to incomplete transcatheter arterial chemoembolization in locally advanced hepatocellular carcinoma. Liver Int 2005;25:1189–1196.
38 Connock M, Round J, Bayliss S, Tubeuf S, Greenheld W, Moore D: Sorafenib for the treatment of advanced hepatocellular carcinoma. Health Technol Assess 2010;14(suppl 1):17–21.

Oncology

Oncology 2013;84(suppl 1):75–81
DOI: 10.1159/000345894

Published online: February 20, 2013

The Prognostic Value of Vascular Endothelial Growth Factor in Hepatocellular Carcinoma for Predicting Metastasis after Curative Resection

Mutsuko Minata[a, e] Kouji H. Harada[b] Masatoshi Kudo[d] Iwao Ikai[c]
Naoshi Nishida[a, d]

[a]Department of Medicine and Clinical Science, Kyoto University Graduate School of Medicine, [b]Kyoto University School of Public Health, and [c]Department of Surgery, National Hospital Organization Kyoto Medical Center, Kyoto, and [d]Department of Gastroenterology and Hepatology, Kinki University Faculty of Medicine, Osakasayama, Japan; [e]Department of Molecular and Cellular Biology, Beckman Research Institute of City of Hope, Duarte, Calif., USA

Key Words

Hepatocellular carcinoma · Vascular endothelial growth factor · E-cadherin · Recurrence

Abstract

Objectives: Hepatocellular carcinoma (HCC) frequently recurs even after curative resection. The purpose of this study was to identify factors predictive for postoperative recurrence of HCC in patients who underwent curative resection using immunohistochemistry. ***Methods:*** Expression of vascular endothelial growth factor (VEGF), E-cadherin and cyclin D1 in HCC tissue were analyzed for 133 HCC patients who underwent curative resection of tumors using immunohistochemical analysis. Relationships of expressions and disease-free survival of HCC were evaluated using univariate and multivariate analyses. ***Results:*** The average period of follow-up of the patients was 6.7 years. Multivariate analyses revealed that only strong expression of VEGF in HCC tissue was significantly associated with metastatic recurrence ($p < 0.001$, hazard ratio, HR, 3.32). ***Conclusions:*** Evaluating VEGF in HCC tissue after surgical resection has predictive value for metastatic HCC recurrence. The ability to risk stratify should improve the treatment strategies after hepatectomy.

Introduction

Postoperative recurrence of hepatocellular carcinoma (HCC) is common and limits long-term survival following otherwise successful surgery [1–3]. Rates of recurrence within 3 years after initial resection have ranged from approximately 60 to 80%, even in HCC tumors smaller than 4 cm or curative resection [4, 5]. A high recurrence rate of HCC is attributed to frequent occurrence of microvascular invasion, occult metastases [6] and multicentric recurrence within a background liver of liver cirrhosis [7]. On the other hand, it was previously demonstrated that metastatic recurrence is associated with angiogenesis and invasiveness of the tumor [8]. Vascular endothelial growth factor (VEGF) is frequently implicated in metastasis by promoting an angiogenic phenotype [9]. Besides, transcriptional inactivation of E-cadherin was shown to occur frequently in tumor progression [10]. From this standpoint, molecular analyses based on genetic profiles of HCC could be useful for predicting the clinical behavior of HCC. However, highly specialized molecular analyses, such as expression microarrays, could not be applicable for clinical setting because of the cost and complexity on analyses. In this study, we investigated an alternative method of molecu-

KARGER

Fax +41 61 306 12 34
E-Mail karger@karger.com
www.karger.com

0030–2414/13/0847–0075$38.00/0

Accessible online at:
www.karger.com/ocl

Naoshi Nishida, MD
Department of Gastroenterology and Hepatology
Kinki University Faculty of Medicine
377-2 Ohno-higashi, Osakasayama, Osaka 589-8511 (Japan)
E-Mail naoshi@med.kindai.ac.jp

lar analysis using immunohistochemical analysis of cancer-related molecules. Specifically, we sought to identify relationships between patterns of recurrence in the expression of VEGF in HCC after curative hepatectomy.

Materials and Methods

Patients

We retrospectively analyzed the relationship between the recurrence of HCCs and clinicopathological parameters in 133 patients who were diagnosed with HCC of stage I or II and underwent curative hepatectomy at Kyoto University Hospital between 1985 and 1993. The mean follow-up period was 6.7 ± 5.2 years (range 0–21) and the patients consisted of 89 men and 44 women with a mean age of 61.4 years. The study was approved by the institutional review board of involved institutions and informed consent was obtained from each patient. The stage of HCC and the curability of surgery were classified according to general rules for the clinical and pathological study of primary liver cancer established by the Liver Cancer Study Group of Japan [11]. After surgery, each patient was monitored every 3 months with serum α-fetoprotein levels and radiological examination of computed tomography or magnetic resonance imaging until September 2008. Abdominal echogram and chest radiograms were also performed every 3 months. Outcome of the patients was classified into 3 groups: recurrence-free (n = 37), multicentric recurrence (n = 22) and metastatic recurrence (n = 74). The patterns of recurrence were assessed morphologically from computed tomography images, angiography, bone scintigrams and pathological findings. Intrahepatic metastatic recurrence was diagnosed as follows: emergence of multiple hypervascular tumors appeared in a localized segment that had contained the original tumor, emergence of a large tumor situated near the original site, emergence of additional smaller tumors in distant parts of the liver [12].

Additional clinicopathological information of the patients are as follows (some data were not available for all patients): status of hepatitis virus, positive for hepatitis B surface antigen (HBsAg; n = 17), positive for hepatitis C virus antibody (HCVAb) or HCV-RNA (n = 77), negative for both HBsAg and HCVAb (n = 5); clinical stage of HCC I (n = 34), II (n = 97); serum alanine aminotransferase (ALT) level ≤80 IU/l (n = 81), >80 IU/l (n = 50); platelet count ($10^3/mm^3$) ≥10 × 10^4 (n = 76), <10 × 10^4 (n = 56); serum α-fetoprotein level ≤400 ng/ml (n = 95), >400 ng/ml (n = 34); histology of noncancerous liver normal (n = 5), chronic hepatitis (n = 35), cirrhosis (n = 89); tumor size <2 cm (n = 47), 2–5 cm (n = 75), >5 cm (n = 11); histological differentiation of HCC well (n = 13), moderate (n = 90), poor (n = 30); vascular invasion positive (n = 2), negative (n = 131). There was no significant correlation between each item of clinicopathological data and patient outcome.

Immunohistochemical Analyses

Immunohistochemical staining for VEGF, E-cadherin and cyclin D1 were performed using the avidin-biotin complex method (Vecstatin ABC kit, Vector Laboratories, Burlingame, Calif., USA). Antibodies used were a rabbit polyclonal antibody for VEGF (Santa Cruz Biotechnology, Santa Cruz, Calif., USA) at a 1:200 dilution, a mouse monoclonal antibody for E-cadherin (Takara Shuzo Co., Shiga, Japan) at a 1:20 dilution and a mouse monoclonal antibody for cyclin D1 (Progen Biotechnik GmbH, Heidelberg, Germany) at a 1:20 dilution. VEGF expression level was scored semi-quantitatively based on staining intensity and distribution using the immunoreactive score (IRS) as described before [13, 14]: IRS = SI (staining intensity) × PP (percentage of positive cells). SI was determined as 0 (negative), 1 (weak), 2 (moderate) and 3 (strong). PP was defined as 0 (negative), 1 (10% positive cells), 2 (11–50% positive cells), 3 (51–80% positive cells) and 4 (more than 80% positive cells). Ten visual fields from different areas of each tumor were used for IRS evaluation. Based on the IRS score, staining intensity was graded into 4 categories of grade 0 (–) (IRS 0–3), grade 1 (+) (IRS 4–6), grade 2 (++) (IRS 7–9) or grade 3 (+++) (IRS 10–12; fig. 1a, b).

To evaluate E-cadherin expression, the immunostaining pattern in normal disease-free liver was used as a positive control. E-cadherin staining was observed at cell-cell borders of all epithelial cells in normal liver; discontinuous or negative membrane staining was defined as abnormal. The approximate intensity of E-cadherin staining in the membrane of each specimen was scored and arranged into three categories: equivalent staining intensity to that of normal hepatic cells was regarded as positive (+), recognizable albeit weaker staining than present in normal cells was classified as weak positive (±) and complete loss of staining was determined as negative (–) (fig. 1c, d).

The expression of cyclin D1 was categorized it as either positive (+) or negative (–). Cyclin D1 expression in cancer was classified as positive staining when more than 30% of tumor cells were positive in high intensity (fig. 1e, f). IHC staining was evaluated independently by two pathologists who were blinded to the patient profiles.

Statistics

Correlations between the expressions of VEGF, E-cadherin and cyclin D1, and clinicopathological features were evaluated using χ^2 tests or Fisher's exact tests. Disease-free survival (DFS) of the patients with each pattern of immunohistochemical staining was estimated using the Kaplan-Meier method and p value of the log-rank tests were calculated. Death was treated as censored at that time. To clarify the relationship between expression of each molecule and metastatic recurrence, we also verified the hazard ratios (HR) of emergence of recurrence within 2 years for each patient group, which were classified according to the intensity of immunohistochemical staining. HR and 95% confidence intervals (95% CI) were calculated with the Cox proportional hazards regression model and each analysis was performed so as to compare different groups (i.e. metastatic recurrence vs. multicentric recurrence, and multicentric recurrence vs. recurrence-free). p values <0.05 were considered statistically significant. The data were managed and analyzed using SAS software (version 9.1, SAS Institute Inc., Cary, N.C., USA).

Results

Correlation between VEGF Expression and Clinical Outcome

VEGF staining was primarily cytoplasmic (fig. 1a, b). The proportion of HCC exhibiting grade 2 or 3 expression of VEGF was significantly higher in patients with

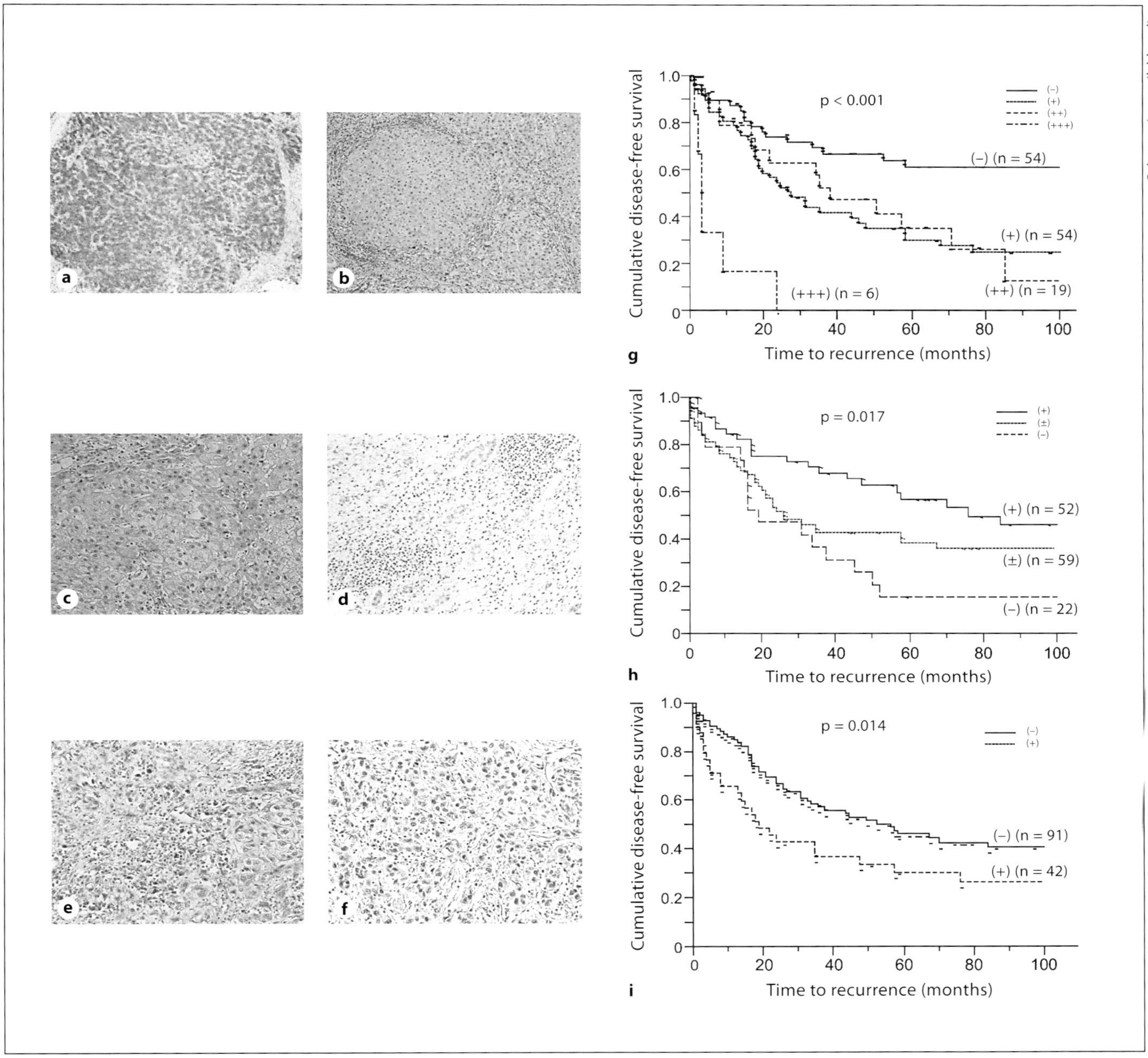

Fig. 1. Immunostaining with a VEGF antibody in HCCs with chronic hepatitis or early cirrhosis: grade 3 (+++) (**a**), negative (–) (**b**). Immunostaining with an E-cadherin antibody in HCCs with chronic hepatitis or early cirrhosis; E-cadherin was observed at cell-cell boundaries: positive (+) (**c**), negative (–) (**d**). Immunostaining with a cyclin D1 antibody in HCCs; cyclin D1 was primarily located in the nucleus: positive (+) (**e**), negative (–) (**f**). **a–f** Original magnification ×200. **g–i** Comparison of cumulative postoperative DFS curves according to intensity. VEGF expression in cancerous tissue (**g**), E-cadherin expression in cancerous tissue (**h**), cyclin D1 expression in cancerous tissue (**i**). Immunostaining intensity was evaluated by the Kaplan-Meier method. All patients with grade 3 (+++) expression of VEGF in cancerous tissues exhibited recurrence within 2 years. The group with grade 1 (+), grade 2 (++) or grade 3 (+++) expression of VEGF in cancerous tissues exhibited higher recurrence rates than those with negative (–) expression of VEGF ($p < 0.001$; log-rank). The group with negative (–) E-cadherin expression in cancerous tissues exhibited shorter periods of DFS than those with weak positive (±) or positive (+) expression. In accordance with reduced E-cadherin expression, the group with reduced E-cadherin expression exhibited higher recurrence rates than those with positive (+) expression of E-cadherin ($p = 0.017$; log-rank). The group with positive (+) expression of cyclin D1 in cancerous tissue exhibited higher recurrence rates than those with negative (–) expression of cyclin D1 ($p = 0.013$; log-rank).

Table 1. Univariate and multivariate analyses

Variable	Univariate			Multivariate		
	HR	95% CI	p	HR	95% CI	p
a *Factors associated with metastatic recurrence (metastatic recurrence vs. multicentric carcinoma and recurrence-free) using univariate and multivariate Cox proportional analysis*						
Platelet count, $10^3/mm^3$						
$\geq 10 \times 10^4$	1.00		–			
$<10 \times 10^4$	1.30	1.03–1.64	0.029			
VEGF expression in HCC tissue						
Negative	1.00		–			
Grade 1	1.54	1.17–2.08	0.002	1.57	1.18–2.13	0.002
Grade 2	1.51	1.05–2.14	0.027	1.52	1.05–2.17	0.027
Grade 3	3.54	2.10–5.60	<0.001	3.32	1.93–5.41	<0.001
E-cadherin expression in HCC tissue						
Positive	1.00		–			
Weak positive	1.29	0.99–1.70	0.056			
Negative	1.58	1.13–2.18	0.008			
Cyclin D1 expression in HCC tissue						
Negative	1.00		–			
Positive	1.34	1.05–1.69	0.019			
b *Factors associated with multicentric carcinoma (multicentric carcinoma vs. recurrence-free) using univariate and multivariate Cox proportional analysis*						
Hepatitis status						
Non-B non-C	1.00		–			
HCV	1.91	1.16–3.57	0.010	1.83	1.11–3.25	0.017
HBV	0.80	0.18–2.08	0.671			
Clinical stage						
I	1.00		–			
II	1.76	1.10–2.78	0.020			
ALT, IU/l						
≤80	1.00		–			
>80	1.58	1.03–2.45	0.035	1.59	1.03–2.48	0.037
Cyclin D1 expression in HCC tissue						
Negative	1.00		–			
Positive	1.46	1.11–1.39	0.18			

p values were calculated for continuous values by ANOVA and for categorical values for the χ^2 test or Fisher's exact test. The patients who had incomplete data were excluded. Non-B non-C denotes negative for HBsAg and HCVAb or HCV-RNA (–); HCV denotes positive for HCVAb or HCV-RNA; HBV denotes positive for HBsAg.

metastatic recurrence (27%; 20/74) than those with multicentric recurrence (9.1%; 2/22) or as recurrence-free (8.1%; 3/37; $p < 0.001$). Notably, all cases of grade 3 VEGF expression were observed exclusively in patients with metastatic recurrence (100%; 6/6).

Table 1 compares HR of metastatic versus multicentric recurrence and recurrence-free, and multicentric recurrence versus recurrence-free. These comparisons were made in relation to clinicopathological data from univariate and multivariate analyses, which were performed to evaluate variables that could affect metastatic recurrence or the emergence of multicentric recurrence after curative surgery. For the onset of metastatic recurrence, the extent of VEGF staining correlated significantly with an increased HR for grade 3 ($p < 0.001$, HR 3.54, 95% CI 2.10–5.60), grade 2 ($p = 0.027$, HR 1.51, 95% CI 1.05–2.14) and grade 1 ($p = 0.002$, HR 1.54, 95% CI 1.17–2.08) by univariate analysis. Multivariate analysis comparing between metastatic recurrence and multicentric recurrence and recurrence-free revealed significantly elevated risk of metastatic recurrence for each grade of VEGF expression (grade 1: $p = 0.002$, HR 1.57, 95% CI 1.18–2.13; grade 2:

$p = 0.027$, HR 1.52, 95% CI 1.05–2.17; grade 3: $p < 0.001$, HR 3.32, 95% CI 1.93–5.41; table 1); however, no significant relationship existed between VEGF expression and multicentric recurrence.

Correlation between E-Cadherin Expression and Clinical Outcome

E-cadherin staining was detected at the cell-cell boundary (fig. 1c, d). Negative E-cadherin expression was observed more frequently in patients with metastatic recurrence (21.6%; 16/74) than in patients with multicentric recurrence (4.5%; 1/22) or recurrence-free (13.5%; 5/37). According to univariate analysis, negative E-cadherin expression indicated increased risk for metastatic recurrence ($p = 0.008$, HR 1.58, 95% CI 1.13–2.18; table 1). However, no significant relationship existed between metastatic recurrence and E-cadherin expression by multivariate analysis. Moreover, there was no significant relationship between E-cadherin expression and multicentric recurrence.

Correlation between Cyclin D1 Expression and Clinical Outcome

Cyclin D1 staining was observed primarily in the nucleus (fig. 1e, f). The positive rate was higher in patients with metastatic recurrence (36.5%; 27/74) than for patients with multicentric recurrence (13.6%; 3/22) or recurrence (32.4%; 12/37), although this was not significant. Univariate analysis demonstrated that expression of cyclin D1 correlated with metastatic recurrence ($p = 0.019$, HR 1.34, 95% CI 1.05–1.69); however, multivariate analysis did not demonstrate a correlation between cyclin D1 expression and metastatic recurrence or multicentric carcinoma (table 1).

Clinical Features of the Patients and Outcome

For metastatic recurrence, low platelet count ($<10 \times 10^4$) was revealed to be the significant correlation in univariate analysis ($p = 0.029$, HR 1.30, 95% CI 1.03–1.64) but not in multivariate analysis. For multicentric recurrence, positivity for HCV ($p = 0.010$, HR 1.91, 95% CI 1.16–3.57), advanced clinical stage of HCC ($p = 0.020$, HR 1.76, 95% CI 1.10–2.78) and serum ALT level (>80; $p = 0.035$, HR 1.58, 95% CI 1.03–2.45) were revealed as the significant relationships by univariate analysis, and the presence of HCV and serum ALT level were selected as independent factors for emergence of multicentric recurrence by multivariate analysis ($p = 0.017$, HR 1.83, 95% CI 1.11–3.25 and $p = 0.037$, HR 1.59, 95% CI 1.03–2.48, respectively; table 1).

DFS, Expression of VEGF, E-Cadherin and Cyclin D1

The median duration of DFS in patients with multicentric recurrence was significantly longer (87.3 ± 56.7 months) than in patients with metastatic recurrence (22.9 ± 20.5 months; $p < 0.001$). The recurrence rate was positively correlated with the extent of VEGF expression ($p < 0.001$; fig. 1g). Notably, all patients with grade 3 VEGF expression occurred recurrence within 2 years and HR of recurrence within 2 years was much higher in grade 3 VEGF expression than the other groups ($p < 0.001$, HR 3.20, 95% CI 1.87–5.17).

Negative or weak E-cadherin expression correlated with shorter periods of DFS, the recurrence rate correlated negatively with the extent of E-cadherin expression ($p = 0.017$; fig. 1h). Moreover, HRs of recurrence within 2 years for negative as well as weak E-cadherin expression were higher than the normal expression group ($p < 0.040$, HR 1.57, 95% CI 1.01–2.42 and $p < 0.02$, HR 1.46, 95% CI 1.04–2.11, respectively). Additionally, positive cyclin D1 expression was correlated with a high rate of recurrence ($p = 0.014$; fig. 1i). HR of recurrence within 2 years for patients with positive cyclin D1 expression was higher than the other groups ($p < 0.005$, HR 1.51, 95% CI 1.13–2.01).

Discussion

Our results confirm the findings of prior studies that evaluated the prognostic value of measuring the expression of cancer-related genes, such as VEGF in HCC [15, 16]. We compared the significance of expression of VEGF, E-cadherin and cyclin D1 on the risk of HCC recurrence after curative resection using immunohistochemical analyses. We found that the extent of VEGF expression in HCC provides the important prognostic information that can be used to evaluate the risk of metastasis following curative hepatic surgery. An interesting dosage-effect of VEGF expression was identified in which HCC patients with grade 3 expression demonstrated the shortest periods of DFS (fig. 1g), which reinforced the notion that angiogenesis plays a pivotal role in metastasis. It is known that metastatic recurrence is early-phase recurrence (within 2 years), whereas those associated with multicentric recurrence contributed to late-phase recurrence (after 2 years) [17], which was consistent with the fact that VEGF expression was associated with metastatic recurrence.

We also found that E-cadherin (reduced expression) and cyclin D1 expression in HCC correlated with metastatic recurrence (table 1). Recent studies suggest that the loss of E-cadherin expression in HCC plays an important role for metastasis by inducing an epithelial-to-mesenchymal transition and disrupting intercellular contacts [18]. Gene expression analysis has also revealed that the loss of E-cadherin contributes to metastatic dissemination by inducing wide-ranging transcriptional and functional changes [19]. On the other hand, overexpression of cyclin D1 reportedly associates with aggressive forms of HCC [20]. Our results suggest that positive expression of cyclin D1 confers an additional growth advantage to the tumor by disrupting cell cycle checkpoints.

Here we have demonstrated the utility of immunohistochemical profiling of VEGF expression in HCC as a predictive biomarker in patients who undergo curative HCC resection. Such analyses can theoretically be performed preoperatively to identify patients most likely to benefit from curative resection. These findings could become important in planning strategies to prevent or reduce HCC recurrence after surgical resection. Recently it has been shown that the treatments to prevent recurrence (including intrahepatic metastasis and multicentric carcinogenesis) are extremely effective for improving the prognosis of HCC patients. For instance, the molecular targeted agent sorafenib, multikinase inhibitors and VEGF inhibitors, significantly prolonged the survival of patients with advanced HCC [21]. Furthermore, another article reported an antibody against placental growth factor (PlGF), a VEGF homolog, which regulates the angiogenic switched in disease, but not in health. αPlGF inhibited growth and metastasis of various tumors [22]. Predicting the recurrence earlier should be important for prolonged prognosis owing to these agents. The IHC expression profiles using HCC tissue revealed high-risk patterns of metastatic recurrence. The results of the current study will contribute to the development of comprehensive adjuvant prevention strategies for postoperative management of HCC.

Disclosure Statement

The authors have no competing interests to declare. This work was supported in part by a grant from the Smoking Research Foundation.

References

1 Zhou XD, Tang ZY, Yang BH, Lin ZY, Ma ZC, Ye SL, Wu ZQ, Fan J, Qin LX, Zheng BH: Experience of 1,000 patients who underwent hepatectomy for small hepatocellular carcinoma. Cancer 2001;91:1479–1486.

2 Nathan H, Schulick RD, Choti MA, Pawlik TM: Predictors of survival after resection of early hepatocellular carcinoma. Ann Surg 2009;249:799–805.

3 Belghiti J, Fuks D: Liver resection and transplantation in hepatocellular carcinoma. Liver Cancer 2012;2:71–82.

4 Nishikawa H, Inuzuka T, Takeda H: Comparison of percutaneous radiofrequency thermal ablation and surgical resection for small hepatocellular carcinoma. BMC Gastroenterol 2011;28:143–154.

5 Choi GH, Kim DH, Kang CM, Kim KS, Choi JS, Lee WJ, Kim BR: Prognostic factors and optimal treatment strategy for intrahepatic nodular recurrence after curative resection of hepatocellular carcinoma. Ann Surg Oncol 2008;15:618–629.

6 Nanashima A, Tobinaga S, Abo T, Kunizaki M, Takeshita H, Hidaka S, Taura N, Ichikawa T, Sawai T, Nakao K, Nagayasu T: Usefulness of sonazoid-ultrasonography during hepatectomy in patients with liver tumors: a preliminary study. J Surg Oncol 2011;103:152–157.

7 Okuda K: Hepatocellular carcinoma: recent progress. Hepatology 1992;15:948–963.

8 Poon RT, Lau CP, Ho JW, Yu WC, Fan ST, Wong J: Tissue factor expression correlates with tumor angiogenesis and invasiveness in human hepatocellular carcinoma. Clin Cancer Res 2003;9:5339–5345.

9 Shibuya M: Vascular endothelial growth factor receptor-1 (VEGFR-1/Flt-1): a dual regulator for angiogenesis. Angiogenesis 2006;9:225–231.

10 Hirohashi S: Inactivation of the E-cadherin-mediated cell adhesion system in human cancers. Am J Pathol 1998;153:333–339.

11 Liver cancer study group of Japan: The general rules for the clinical and pathological study of primary liver cancer. Jpn J Surg 1989;19:98–129.

12 Ikeda K, Arase Y, Kobayashi M, Saitoh S, Someya T, Hosaka T, Suzuki Y, Suzuki F, Tsubota A, Akuta N, Kumada H: Significance of multicentric cancer recurrence after potentially curative ablation of hepatocellular carcinoma: a longterm cohort study of 892 patients with viral cirrhosis. J Gastroenterol 2003;38:865–876.

13 Chui X, Egami H, Yamashita J, Kurizaki T, Ohmachi H, Yamamoto S, Ogawa M: Immunohistochemical expression of the c-kit proto-oncogene product in human malignant and non-malignant breast tissues. Br J Cancer 1996;73:1233–1236.

14 Friedrichs K, Gluba S, Eidtmann H, Jonat W: Overexpression of p53 and prognosis in breast cancer. Cancer 1993;72:3641–3647.

15 Yang JC, Teng CF, Wu HC, Tsai HW, Chuang HC, Tsai TF, Hsu YH, Huang W, Wu LW, Su IJ: Enhanced expression of vascular endothelial growth factor-A in ground glass hepatocytes and its implication in hepatitis B virus hepatocarcinogenesis. Hepatology 2009;49:1962–1971.

16 Schoenleber SJ, Kurtz DM, Talwalkar JA, Roberts LR, Gores GJ: Prognostic role of vascular endothelial growth factor in hepatocellular carcinoma: systematic review and meta-analysis. Br J Cancer 2009;100:1385–1392.
17 Imamura H, Matsuyama Y, Tanaka E, Ohkubo T, Hasegawa K, Miyagawa S, Sugawara Y, Minagawa M, Takayama T, Kawasaki S, Makuuchi M: Risk factors contributing to early and late phase intrahepatic recurrence of hepatocellular carcinoma after hepatectomy. J Hepatol 2003;38:200–207.
18 Schmalhofer O, Brabletz S, Brabletz T: E-cadherin, β-catenin, and ZEB1 in malignant progression of cancer. Cancer Metastasis Rev 2009;28:151–166.
19 Onder TT, Gupta PB, Mani SA, Yang J, Lander ES, Weinberg RA: Loss of E-cadherin promotes metastasis via multiple downstream transcriptional pathways. Cancer Res 2008;68:3645–3654.
20 Nishida N, Fukuda Y, Komeda T, Kita R, Sando T, Furukawa M, Amenomori M, Shibagaki I, Nakao K, Ikenaga M, et al: Amplification and overexpression of the cyclin D1 gene in aggressive human hepatocellular carcinoma. Cancer Res 1994;54:3107–3110.
21 Kudo M: Adjuvant therapy after curative treatment for hepatocellular carcinoma. Oncology 2011;81(suppl 1):50–55.
22 Fischer C, Jonckx B, Mazzone M, Zacchigna S, Loges S, Pattarini L, Chorianopoulos E, Liesenborghs L, Koch M, De Mol M, Autiero M, Wyns S, Plaisance S, Moons L, van Rooijen N, Giacca M, Stassen JM, Dewerchin M, Collen D, Carmeliet P: Anti-PlGF inhibits growth of VEGF(R)-inhibitor-resistant tumors without affecting healthy vessels. Cell 2007;131:463–475.

Oncology

Oncology 2013;84(suppl 1):82–87
DOI: 10.1159/000345895

Published online: February 20, 2013

Quantification of Tumor DNA in Serum and Vascular Invasion of Human Hepatocellular Carcinoma

Naoshi Nishida[a, b] Tadaaki Arizumi[a] Masahiro Takita[a] Tomoyuki Nagai[a] Satoshi Kitai[a] Norihisa Yada[a] Satoru Hagiwara[a] Tatsuo Inoue[a] Yasunori Minami[a] Kazuomi Ueshima[a] Toshiharu Sakurai[a] Hiroshi Ida[b] Masatoshi Kudo[a]

[a]Department of Gastroenterology and Hepatology, Kinki University Faculty of Medicine, Osakasayama, and
[b]Department of Gastroenterology and Hepatology, Kyoto University Graduate School of Medicine, Kyoto, Japan

Key Words

Hepatocellular carcinoma · Tumor suppressor gene · DNA methylation · Epigenetics · Molecular diagnosis

Abstract

Objectives: Hepatocellular carcinoma (HCC) is one of the common cancers worldwide. Accurate diagnosis of tumor progression is critical for the appropriate management of HCC. Here, we established a sensitive assay to detect and quantify tumor-derived DNA in the serum of HCC patients. ***Methods:*** Aberrant methylation of the *APC* gene was quantified in 23 HCC patients and 8 healthy volunteers using 100 μl of serum. For sensitive detection and accurate quantification of tumor DNA, we combined seminested polymerase chain reaction (PCR) with TaqMan PCR, which could amplify the *APC* gene regardless of the methylation status and detect the methylated and unmethylated sequences separately. The ratio of methylated to unmethylated sequences was quantified. ***Results:*** The methylated *APC* gene was detected in all HCC patients examined, but no healthy volunteers showed amplification of methylated sequences in serum. HCC patients with portal vein thrombosis showed a significantly higher methylated to unmethylated *APC* gene ratio in serum than those without portal vein thrombosis ($p = 0.0029$). ***Conclusions:*** Considering the strong association between the ratio of the methylated to unmethylated *APC* sequences in serum and the presence of portal vein thrombosis, methylation status of *APC* sequences could be a promising marker for improving HCC management.

Introduction

Hepatocellular carcinoma (HCC) is one of the most common cancers in the world, and infection with hepatitis B virus or hepatitis C virus is a critical risk for the emergence of this type of malignancy. The number of HCC patients is expected to increase after recent studies revealed that several types of common metabolic disorder such as diabetes mellitus and obesity could also act as important factors for accelerating HCC development [1]. Surgical treatment [2], radiofrequency ablation [3] and trance catheter arterial chemoembolization [4] are well-known major treatment options; however, the prognosis of advanced HCC is unsatisfactory because of the lack of effective therapeutic alternatives [1].

KARGER

Fax +41 61 306 12 34
E-Mail karger@karger.com
www.karger.com

0030–2414/13/0847–0082$38.00/0

Accessible online at:
www.karger.com/ocl

Naoshi Nishida, MD
Department of Gastroenterology and Hepatology
Kinki University Faculty of Medicine
377-2 Ohno-higashi, Osakasayama, Osaka 589-8511 (Japan)
E-Mail naoshi@med.kindai.ac.jp

Recent advancements in the study of molecular targeted agents such as sorafenib have resulted in improved survival rates of patients with advanced HCC and increased time to progression, even in cases that failed to achieve tumor regression [5]. However, estimation of this type of tumor response, or response to 'dormant therapy', is sometimes difficult because the lack of tumor regression identified through imaging studies could be regarded as treatment failure, even in cases of stable disease with prolonged time to progression, which could be a benefit of treatment with sorafenib. Imaging studies are also inadequate for estimating a total tumor burden because the advanced tumors are usually associated with multiple small metastatic lesions. Therefore, in addition to imaging studies, conventional tumor markers such as α-fetoproteins (AFP) and des-γ-carboxy prothrombin (DCP) have been examined to evaluate the dynamics of tumor volume during treatment [6]. Although a combination of AFP and DCP reportedly improved the sensitivity of diagnosing HCC, a considerable number of HCC patients failed to show an increase in tumor marker levels [7]. In these patients, conventional tumor markers were not useful for the estimation of tumor response during the course of HCC treatment.

Generally, the molecular pathogenesis of cancer development involves multiple genetic and epigenetic aberrations, which lead to activation of oncogenes and inactivation of tumor suppressor genes (TSGs) [8]. Recent reports have suggested that quantification of circulating mutant genes from tumor cells could be useful in assessing the tumor dynamics of colon cancer during treatment and that this personalized genetic approach could be generally applied to patients with other types of cancer [9]. So far, we have intensively analyzed genetic and epigenetic alterations in oncogenes and TSGs in human HCC tissues [10–13]. Although recurrent genetic alterations of individual genes are not frequent, epigenetic alterations such as methylation of the promoter of TSGs occur far more frequently. In particular, we found that abnormal methylation of the promoter of the adenomatous polyposis coli *(APC)* gene was seen in a majority of HCC tissues, and the methylation level of the *APC* gene was considerably different between HCC tissue and the corresponding noncancerous liver tissue [14].

In this study, we developed a sensitive assay for the quantification of cancer-specific DNA in serum of HCC patients, based on the methylated *APC* gene. We explored the possible diagnostic value of this tumor-specific DNA alteration for tumor detection. We found the amount of the methylated *APC* gene in serum to be strongly correlated with vascular invasion of HCC. In addition, quantification of this epigenetic alteration could be a powerful tool to estimate the aggressiveness of the tumor as well as tumor dynamics during the treatment of HCC.

Materials and Methods

Patients

Twenty-three HCC patients and 8 healthy volunteers were analyzed to quantify promoter methylation of the *APC* gene using serum DNA. The clinical backgrounds of the HCC patients were as follows: median age was 71 years (25th and 75th percentiles: 66 and 73); 14 were male and 9 were female, and 4 were hepatitis B virus surface antigen (HBsAg) positive, 13 were hepatitis C virus antibody (HCVAb) positive, 2 were positive for both HBsAg and HCVAb, and 4 were negative for both. Among 23 patients, 7 showed portal vein invasion and 19 showed multiple HCCs (2 or more) on contrast enhanced-computed tomography. Three HCC patients were classified as stage 1, 2 as stage 2, 11 as stage 3 and 7 as stage 4. Median serum AFP and DCP levels were 76 ng/ml (25th and 75th percentiles: 21 and 778) and 307 mAU/ml (25 and 1,169), respectively. Informed consent was obtained from each patient and the study was approved by the institutional review board of the involved institution.

Quantification of Methylation Levels in Serum DNA

DNA was extracted from 100 μl of serum using the DNA Extractor SP Kit according to the manufacturer's protocol (Wako Pure Chemical Industries Ltd., Osaka, Japan). The serum DNA samples were subjected to bisulfite treatment using the EpiTect™ Bisulfite kit (QIAGEN Inc., Valencia, Calif., USA). We selected the methylated *APC* gene as a target for the detection of tumor DNA because our previous analysis indicated aberrant methylation of the *APC* gene in 84% of HCC cases [14, 15]. In addition, the difference in the methylation level between HCC and noncancerous liver tissues was most prominent in the promoter of the *APC* gene among the CpG loci examined. HCC tissues showed a high level of methylation, but methylation was extremely low in noncancerous tissues [14, 15]. Thus, the methylation level of this gene made it an ideal candidate for quantification of tumor-derived DNA in serum of HCC patients in the context of minimizing false-positive and false-negative errors. For the quantification of methylated *APC* genes, the ratio of amount of the methylated to unmethylated *APC* gene was determined using the StepOne™ real-time detection system (Applied Biosystems, Foster City, Calif., USA). In order to increase the sensitivity for detecting small amounts of methylated DNA, we used semi-nested PCR with setting TaqMan probes for the detection of inner PCR products that are specific for the methylated or unmethylated *APC* gene (fig. 1a). These primers and probes were designed to amplify the promoter of the *APC* gene. The PCR primers and probes used in this assay were as follows: forward outer PCR primer, 5′-GGTTATGTGTGTTTATATTTAGTTAATTGGTG-3′ and reverse outer PCR primer, 5′-AAATACAAACCAAAACACTCCCC-3′. The inner forward nested-PCR primer and TaqMan probe for detecting the methylated *APC* gene pro-

Fig. 1. Sensitive detection and quantification of the ratio of methylated to unmethylated *APC* genes. **a** Heminested PCR for the methylated and unmethylated *APC* genes. Using outer primers, which do not contain a CpG site, the *APC* gene was amplified regardless of methylation status. However, methylated and unmethylated *APC* genes can be detected separately by using the inner heminested primer and TaqMan probe specific for the methylated and unmethylated sequences, respectively. A filled circle and an empty circle represent a methylated and unmethylated CpG site, respectively. Amplification curve (**b**) and standard curve (**c**) for PCR of the methylated and unmethylated *APC* genes; the efficiency of PCR amplification of the methylated and unmethylated *APC* genes was almost equal.

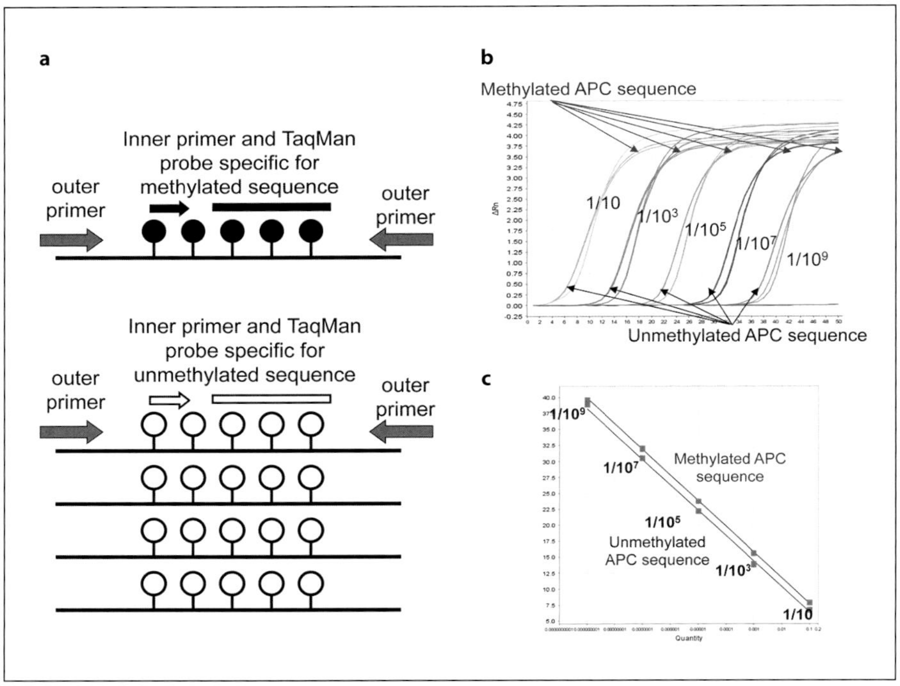

Color version available online

moter were 5′-TTATATGTCGGTTACGTGCGTTTATAT-3′ and FAM-CCCGTCGAAAACCCGCCGATTA-MBG, respectively. The inner PCR forward primer and TaqMan probe specific for the unmethylated promoter were 5′-GGTTATGTGTGTTTATATTTAGTTAATTGGTG-3′ and FAM-TTCCCATCAAAAAC-MGB, respectively. We expected that both methylated and unmethylated promoters would be equally amplified on using the outer primer pairs, which do not contain the CpG sequence. However, the methylated and unmethylated promoters would be quantified separately on using the specific inner primer pairs and TaqMan probes for methylated or unmethylated DNA (fig. 1a). The PCR was performed according to the manufacturer's protocol using TaqMan® Fast Universal PCR Master Mix (Applied Biosystems). A standard curve for each assay was generated by the serial dilution of bisulfite-treated CpGenome™ Universal Methylated DNA (Chemicon International Inc., Temecula, Calif., USA). The ratio of amount of the methylated to unmethylated *APC* gene was calculated using the StepOne™ real-time detection system (Applied Biosystems).

Statistical Analysis

The Wilcoxon rank-sum test was applied to compare the differences in the ratio of methylated to unmethylated *APC* gene levels between any 2 categorical variables of clinical factors. Continuous variables such as age, serum AFP levels and serum DCP levels were each categorized into 2 subgroups: <70 or ≥ 70 years, <100 or ≥ 100 ng/ml, and <400 or >400 mAU/ml, respectively. All p values were two-sided and $p < 0.05$ was considered statistically significant. All statistical analyses were performed using JMP version 9.0 software (SAS Institute Inc., Cary, N.C., USA).

Results

Amplification of the Methylated and Unmethylated APC Genes

Using the sensitive assay, a combined seminested and real-time PCR-detection system, we successfully amplified both the methylated and unmethylated *APC* gene from serum DNA. Figure 1b, c shows the amplification and standard curve of the methylated and unmethylated gene products, respectively. The 2 standard curves for the amplification of the methylated and unmethylated genes revealed that amplification efficiency should be similar for the 2 heminested PCR products of the methylated and unmethylated genes. The serum DNA of 8 healthy volunteers showed amplification of the unmethylated gene, but no amplification of the methylated gene. In contrast, serum DNA samples from all 23 HCC patients showed amplification of the methylated as well as the unmethylated gene, and we were able to calculate the ratio of methylated to unmethylated DNA in 20 of 23 samples. The mean value was 9% (25th and 75th percentiles: 8.0 and 18.8%). For 3 of 23 serum DNA samples, the ratio of methylated to unmethylated DNA could not be determined because of the low level (less than 1%) of the methylated APC allele.

Table 1. Association between the ratio of the methylated to unmethylated *APC* gene in serum DNA and clinical background of HCC patients

Clinical background (number of cases)	Mean ratio, % (25–75th percentiles)	p value
Age		
<70 years (10)	11 (7–18.25)	0.2256
≥70 years (10)	5.5 (3.75–23.5)	
Gender		
Male (11)	11 (7–18)	0.2697
Female (9)	5 (3.5–23)	
Viral status		
HBV (4)	21 (11.25–27)	0.2626
HCV (11)	7 (4–19)	
HBV and HCV (2)	8 (5–11)	
Virus negative (3)	7 (2–13)	
Tumors, n		
<2 (4)	11 (5.5–25)	0.3066
≥2 (16)	8 (4.5–18.25)	
Maximal tumor size		
<3 cm (10)	9 (6.25–12.5)	1.0000
≥3 cm (10)	9 (4.25–21.25)	
Portal vein thrombosis		
Presence (7)	19 (11–28)	0.0029*
Absence (13)	6 (4–10)	
Serum AFP level		
<100 ng/ml (8)	7 (3.25–10.5)	0.1527
≥100 ng/ml (12)	12 (6.25–21.25)	
Serum DCP level		
<400 mAU/ml (11)	9 (5–22)	0.7320
≥400 mAU/ml (9)	7 (5–2)	

Three patients who showed a ratio of less than 1% were excluded from the analysis. Continuous variables of age, serum AFP and DCP level were categorized into two subgroups of <70 or ≥70 years, <100 or ≥100 ng/ml, and <400 or ≥400 mAU/ml, respectively. p values calculated by the Wilcoxon rank-sum test. * $p < 0.05$.

Relationship between the Ratio of Methylated to Unmethylated Gene Sequences and Clinical Backgrounds of HCC Patients

Table 1 shows the relationship between the ratio of the methylated to unmethylated *APC* genes in serum and the clinical background of each HCC patient. Clinical background variables such as age, gender and status of hepatitis virus were not associated with this ratio. In addition, no significant association was noted between the levels of conventional tumor markers AFP and DCP and the degree of the methylated *APC* gene. In contrast, although the factors of tumor size and number did not affect the ratio of the methylated to unmethylated genes, HCC patients with portal vein thrombosis showed a significantly higher degree of the methylated *APC* gene in serum DNA ($p = 0.0029$ by the Wilcoxon rank-sum test; table 1). The mean values of the ratio of methylated to unmethylated genes in patients with and without portal vein thrombosis were 19% (25th and 75th percentiles: 11 and 28%) and 6% (4 and 10%), respectively (table 1).

Discussion

HCC is one of the most common malignancies worldwide, and the overall prevalence of the at-risk population is still growing. Although the definitive molecular pathogenesis of HCC still needs to be clarified, several reports describe different forms of genetic and epigenetic alterations in HCC [8]. Recent genome-wide analysis of human HCC tissues revealed that a variety of genes harbored several types of genetic alterations; however, the frequency of alteration types in individual cancer-related genes was low compared with epigenetic changes such as promoter methylation of TSGs [8, 16]. Therefore, we hypothesized that the evolution and progression of this disease may involve epigenetic alterations, which could be a target for the detection of tumor DNA in serum.

So far, many studies have tried to detect tumor-associated aberrant methylation of TSGs in the circulation of patients with HCC. Wong et al. [17] reported that the methylated *CDKN2A* sequence was found in the serum of HCC patients, and that methylation was evident in the *CDKN2A* gene in the tumor. More recently, it was reported that the quantification of tumor-specific methylated genes in the serum of HCC patients could be applied to predict disease-free survival after hepatectomy [18], and as a valuable biomarker for early detection in populations at high risk of HCC [19]. These results suggest that circulating tumor-derived DNA could be detected using tumor-associated DNA methylation changes and that this approach may have implications for the noninvasive detection of HCCs as well as the prediction of aggressive tumor behavior.

Treatment of advanced HCC is still unsatisfactory because of high tumor recurrence rates. In particular, invasion into the portal vein is a characteristic feature of advanced HCC, which limits treatment options. However, advances in molecular targeted therapy, such as the use of sorafenib, can possibly play an important role in the treatment of this refractory tumor, especially a tumor with metastasis or portal vein thrombosis [5]. Predictive biomarkers for sorafenib treatment are still undetermined, making early detection of vascular invasion critical in determining the timing of the administration of sorafenib [20]. Consequently, the results obtained from our study are clinically important because we found a significant association between increase of methylated *APC* gene in serum and the presence of portal vein thrombosis. As tumor-derived DNA in serum should be a result of the moving out of DNA from HCC tissue to circulation [9], the results of this study are reasonable; high levels of methylated sequences of tumor DNA were observed in HCC patients, especially in those with vascular invasion. In addition, the results indicated that the ratio of methylated to unmethylated DNA did not significantly correlate with the levels of other conventional tumor markers such as AFP and DCP. Because these conventional markers are also associated with tumor growth [6], the combination of tumor-derived methylated DNA measurement and AFP and DCP level evaluation could provide a powerful tool for early detection and prediction of portal vein thrombosis in HCC patients [21]. This information can be applied to HCC management in the context of treatment selection [20]. Furthermore, measurements of circulating tumor DNA can possibly be applied to reliably monitor tumor dynamics in patients undergoing cancer therapy [18]. Reduction in tumor-derived DNA levels occurred faster than the reduction in conventional tumor marker levels after effective treatment [9], so we concluded that the measurement of circulating tumor DNA, such as the methylated *APC* sequence, in the serum of HCC patients could be critical for early determination of therapy effectiveness [22]. This is of importance because the establishment of second-line therapy for refractory HCC cases is currently under investigation.

In this study, we established a novel assay for the sensitive detection and quantification of tumor-derived DNA in the peripheral blood of HCC patients based on the aberrant methylation of the *APC* gene. We successfully quantified tumor DNA in the peripheral blood of these patients using small amounts of serum. Our previous study revealed that methylation of the *APC* gene was detected in a majority of HCC cases and could discriminate HCC from noncancerous liver tissue. Therefore, the methylated *APC* sequence is an ideal target for the detection of tumorous DNA in peripheral blood. Considering the strong association between the ratio of methylated to unmethylated *APC* sequences in serum and the presence of portal vein thrombosis in HCC, quantification of the methylated sequence of the *APC* gene could be a promising approach for the management of advanced HCC.

Disclosure Statement

The authors have no competing interests to declare. This work was supported in part by a grant from the Smoking Research Foundation.

References

1 Kim DY, Han K-H: Epidemiology and surveillance of hepatocellular carcinoma. Liver Cancer 2012;1:2–14.
2 Belghiti J, Fuks D: Liver resection and transplantation in hepatocellular carcinoma. Liver Cancer 2012;1:71–82.
3 Kuang M, Wang Y, Jiang C, Xie XY, Lu MD: A precise safety margin of 1.0 cm is required for best local efficacy of radiofrequency ablation of hepatocellular carcinoma: assessment with a novel three dimensional reconstruction software. Liver Cancer 2012;1:125.
4 Lencioni R: Chemoembolization in patients with hepatocellular carcinoma. Liver Cancer 2012;1:41–50.
5 Llovet JM, Ricci S, Mazzaferro V, Hilgard P, Gane E, Blanc JF, de Oliveira AC, Santoro A, Raoul JL, Forner A, Schwartz M, Porta C, Zeuzem S, Bolondi L, Greten TF, Galle PR, Seitz JF, Borbath I, Haussinger D, Giannaris T, Shan M, Moscovici M, Voliotis D, Bruix J: Sorafenib in advanced hepatocellular carcinoma. N Engl J Med 2008;359:378–390.
6 Koike Y, Shiratori Y, Sato S, Obi S, Teratani T, Imamura M, Yoshida H, Shiina S, Omata M: Des-gamma-carboxy prothrombin as a useful predisposing factor for the development of portal venous invasion in patients with hepatocellular carcinoma: a prospective analysis of 227 patients. Cancer 2001;91: 561–569.
7 Lok AS, Sterling RK, Everhart JE, Wright EC, Hoefs JC, Di Bisceglie AM, Morgan TR, Kim HY, Lee WM, Bonkovsky HL, Dienstag JL: Des-γ-carboxy prothrombin and α-fetoprotein as biomarkers for the early detection of hepatocellular carcinoma. Gastroenterology 2010;138:493–502.
8 Nishida N, Goel A: Genetic and epigenetic signatures in human hepatocellular carcinoma: a systematic review. Curr Genomics 2011;12:130–137.
9 Diehl F, Schmidt K, Choti MA, Romans K, Goodman S, Li M, Thornton K, Agrawal N, Sokoll L, Szabo SA, Kinzler KW, Vogelstein B, Diaz LA Jr: Circulating mutant DNA to assess tumor dynamics. Nat Med 2008;14: 985–990.
10 Nishida N, Fukuda Y, Kokuryu H, Toguchida J, Yandell DW, Ikenega M, Imura H, Ishizaki K: Role and mutational heterogeneity of the p53 gene in hepatocellular carcinoma. Cancer Res 1993;53:368–372.
11 Nishida N, Fukuda Y, Komeda T, Kita R, Sando T, Furukawa M, Amenomori M, Shibagaki I, Nakao K, Ikenaga M, et al: Amplification and overexpression of the cyclin d1 gene in aggressive human hepatocellular carcinoma. Cancer Res 1994;54: 3107–3110.
12 Nishida N: Impact of hepatitis virus and aging on DNA methylation in human hepatocarcinogenesis. Histol Histopathol 2010;25: 647–654.
13 Nishida N, Kudo M, Nagasaka T, Ikai I, Goel A: Characteristic patterns of altered DNA methylation predict emergence of human hepatocellular carcinoma. Hepatology 2012; 56:994–1003.

14 Nishida N, Nagasaka T, Nishimura T, Ikai I, Boland CR, Goel A: Aberrant methylation of multiple tumor suppressor genes in aging liver, chronic hepatitis, and hepatocellular carcinoma. Hepatology 2008;47:908–918.
15 Nishida N, Nishimura T, Nagasaka T, Ikai I, Goel A, Boland CR: Extensive methylation is associated with beta-catenin mutations in hepatocellular carcinoma: evidence for two distinct pathways of human hepatocarcinogenesis. Cancer Res 2007;67:4586–4594.
16 Fujimoto A, Totoki Y, Abe T, Boroevich KA, Hosoda F, Nguyen HH, Aoki M, Hosono N, Kubo M, Miya F, Arai Y, Takahashi H, Shirakihara T, Nagasaki M, Shibuya T, Nakano K, Watanabe-Makino K, Tanaka H, Nakamura H, Kusuda J, Ojima H, Shimada K, Okusaka T, Ueno M, Shigekawa Y, Kawakami Y, Arihiro K, Ohdan H, Gotoh K, Ishikawa O, Ariizumi S, Yamamoto M, Yamada T, Chayama K, Kosuge T, Yamaue H, Kamatani N, Miyano S, Nakagama H, Nakamura Y, Tsunoda T, Shibata T, Nakagawa H: Whole-genome sequencing of liver cancers identifies etiological influences on mutation patterns and recurrent mutations in chromatin regulators. Nat Genet 2012;44:760–764.
17 Wong IH, Lo YM, Zhang J, Liew CT, Ng MH, Wong N, Lai PB, Lau WY, Hjelm NM, Johnson PJ: Detection of aberrant p16 methylation in the plasma and serum of liver cancer patients. Cancer Res 1999;59:71–73.
18 Wong IH, Zhang J, Lai PB, Lau WY, Lo YM: Quantitative analysis of tumor-derived methylated *p16ink4a* sequences in plasma, serum, and blood cells of hepatocellular carcinoma patients. Clin Cancer Res 2003;9: 1047–1052.
19 Zhang YJ, Wu HC, Shen J, Ahsan H, Tsai WY, Yang HI, Wang LY, Chen SY, Chen CJ, Santella RM: Predicting hepatocellular carcinoma by detection of aberrant promoter methylation in serum DNA. Clin Cancer Res 2007;13:2378–2384.
20 Llovet JM, Pena CE, Lathia CD, Shan M, Meinhardt G, Bruix J: Plasma biomarkers as predictors of outcome in patients with advanced hepatocellular carcinoma. Clin Cancer Res 2012;18:2290–2300.
21 Iizuka N, Oka M, Sakaida I, Moribe T, Miura T, Kimura N, Tamatsukuri S, Ishitsuka H, Uchida K, Terai S, Yamashita S, Okita K, Sakata K, Karino Y, Toyota J, Ando E, Ide T, Sata M, Tsunedomi R, Tsutsui M, Iida M, Tokuhisa Y, Sakamoto K, Tamesa T, Fujita Y, Hamamoto Y: Efficient detection of hepatocellular carcinoma by a hybrid blood test of epigenetic and classical protein markers. Clin Chim Acta 2011;412:152–158.
22 Kawakami K, Brabender J, Lord RV, Groshen S, Greenwald BD, Krasna MJ, Yin J, Fleisher AS, Abraham JM, Beer DG, Sidransky D, Huss HT, Demeester TR, Eads C, Laird PW, Ilson DH, Kelsen DP, Harpole D, Moore MB, Danenberg KD, Danenberg PV, Meltzer SJ: Hypermethylated APC DNA in plasma and prognosis of patients with esophageal adenocarcinoma. J Natl Cancer Inst 2000;92:1805–1811.

Oncology

Oncology 2013;84(suppl 1):88–92
DOI: 10.1159/000345896

Published online: February 20, 2013

Expression of E-Cadherin and Vascular Endothelial Growth Factor in Noncancerous Liver Is Associated with Recurrence of Hepatocellular Carcinoma after Curative Resection

Mutsuko Minata[a, e] Masatoshi Kudo[d] Kouji H. Harada[b] Iwao Ikai[c]
Naoshi Nishida[a, d]

[a]Department of Medicine and Clinical Science, Kyoto University Graduate School of Medicine, [b]Kyoto University School of Public Health, and [c]Department of Surgery, National Hospital Organization Kyoto Medical Center, Kyoto, and [d]Department of Gastroenterology and Hepatology, Kinki University Faculty of Medicine, Osakasayama, Japan; [e]Department of Molecular and Cellular Biology, Beckman Research Institute of City of Hope, Duarte, Calif., USA

Key Words
Hepatocellular carcinoma · E-cadherin · Recurrence · Vascular endothelial growth factor · Metastasis

Abstract
Objectives: Hepatocellular carcinoma (HCC) frequently recurs even after curative resection. The purpose of this study was to examine how background liver affects postoperative recurrence of HCC that underwent curative resection using expression of cancer-related molecules in the adjacent noncancerous liver of HCC patients. ***Methods:*** We examined expression of E-cadherin and vascular endothelial growth factor in noncancerous liver tissues of 133 HCC patients who underwent curative resection of tumors using immunohistochemical analysis. Associations between expressions of these molecules and disease-free survival of HCC were analyzed using the Kaplan-Meier method. ***Results:*** The average period of follow-up of the patients was 6.7 years. Multivariate analyses revealed that low platelet count and negative expression of E-cadherin in adjacent noncancerous liver were significantly associated with metastatic recurrence [$p = 0.017$, hazard ratio (HR) = 1.31 for low platelet count, and $p = 0.009$, HR = 1.43 for negative expression of E-cadherin, respectively]. ***Conclusions:*** Expression levels of E-cadherin in adjacent noncancerous liver after surgical resection was associated with metastatic HCC recurrence later on. Analysis of E-cadherin expression should provide important information for predicting recurrence after curative resection of HCC.

Introduction

Despite significant advances in early detection and therapy for hepatocellular carcinoma (HCC), recurrence rate of this tumor is still high and long-term survival remains poor [1]. Recurrence of HCC can be divided into metastasis and multicentric recurrence [2]. However, so far, more than 90% of cancer-related deaths are attributed to the recurrence of tumor metastasis [3]. In addition, recent studies have revealed that epithelial-mesenchymal transition (EMT) is critically involved in invasion and metastasis in cancer, and loss of E-cadherin expression reportedly plays a critical role for phenotype of EMT [4]. Besides, it has also been reported that vascular endothelial growth factor (VEGF)-responsive precursor cells are necessary for neovascularization in the premetastatic

KARGER

Fax +41 61 306 12 34
E-Mail karger@karger.com
www.karger.com

0030–2414/13/0847–0088$38.00/0

Accessible online at:
www.karger.com/ocl

Naoshi Nishida, MD
Department of Gastroenterology and Hepatology
Kinki University Faculty of Medicine
377-2 Ohno-higashi, Osakasayama, Osaka 589-8511 (Japan)
E-Mail naoshi@med.kindai.ac.jp

niche [5]. From this standpoint, analyses of E-cadherin and VEGF based on genetic profiles in the background liver of HCC patients should be important for predicting the biological behavior of HCC. We investigated the relationships between patterns of recurrence and the expression of E-cadherin or VEGF in noncancerous liver tissue of HCC patients after curative hepatectomy using an immunohistochemical analysis.

Material and Methods

Patients

The tissue samples were collected from 133 HCC patients who were consecutively treated with surgery for primary HCC between 1985 and 1993 at Kyoto University Hospital. We specifically selected and focused on the patients who curatively resected of HCC with stage I or II and retrospectively analyzed the correlation between the recurrence of HCC and their clinicopathological parameters (over a median follow-up period of 6.7 ± 5.2 years). This study was performed based on the consent of the institutional review board of involved institutions and informed consent was obtained from each patient. We classified the stage of HCC and the surgical curability according to the criteria of general rules established by the Liver Cancer Study Group of Japan for the clinical and pathological study of primary liver cancer [6]. Every 3 months until September 2008, all patients were followed up with regular monitoring for serum α-fetoprotein level, and computerized tomographic (CT) scan or magnetic resonance imaging (MRI) of the liver in addition to abdominal echogram and chest radiograms. The diagnosis of recurrence was based on CT or angiography and, if necessary, bone scintigram was performed. Pathological findings of recurrent tumor tissues were also taken into consideration if available. Intrahepatic metastatic recurrence was diagnosed as follows: emergence of multiple hypervascular tumors appeared in a localized segment that had contained the original tumor, emergence of a large tumor situated near the original site and emergence of additional smaller tumors in distant parts of the liver [7]. Finally, the outcome of the patients was categorized into 3 groups of recurrence-free (n = 37), multicentric recurrence (n = 22) and metastatic recurrence (n = 74).

Additional clinicopathological information of the patients are as follows: sex, male (n = 89), female (n = 44) with a mean age of 61.4 years; status of hepatitis virus, positive for hepatitis B virus antigen (n = 17), positive for hepatitis C virus antibody or hepatitis C virus RNA (n = 77), negative for both hepatitis B virus antigen and hepatitis C virus (n = 5); clinical stage of HCC, I (n = 34), II (n = 97); serum alanine aminotransferase (ALT) level ≤80 IU/l (n = 81), >80 IU/l (n = 50); platelet count ($10^3/mm^3$) $\geq 10 \times 10^4$ (n = 76), $<10 \times 10^4$ (n = 56); serum α-fetoprotein level ≤400 ng/ml (n = 95), >400 ng/ml (n = 34); histology of noncancerous liver, normal (n = 5), chronic hepatitis (n = 35), cirrhosis (n = 89); tumor size <2 cm (n = 47), 2–5 cm (n = 75), >5 cm (n = 11); histological differentiation of HCC, well (n = 13), moderate (n = 90), poor (n = 30); vascular invasion, positive (n = 2), negative (n = 131). No significant correlation was observed between each clinicopathological category and patient outcome.

Immunohistochemical Analyses

We performed immunohistochemical staining for E-cadherin and VEGF using the avidin-biotin complex method (Vecstatin ABC kit, Vector Laboratories, Burlingame, Calif., USA). Antibodies were: E-cadherin, a rabbit polyclonal (Takara Shuzo Co., Shiga, Japan) at a 1:20 dilution and VEGF, a mouse monoclonal (Santa Cruz Biotechnology, Santa Cruz, Calif., USA) at a 1:200 dilution. E-cadherin staining was observed at cell-cell borders of all epithelial cells in normal liver, discontinuous or negative membrane staining was defined as abnormal. The E-cadherin expression patterns were divided into three groups as follows: (1) positive (+), E-cadherin staining was similar to that of normal hepatic cells; (2) weak positive (±), staining was weaker than present in normal cells; (3) negative (–), complete loss of staining was discerned. VEGF staining was primarily cytoplasmic, the percentage of positive cells was semi-quantitatively counted based on staining intensity and distribution using the immunoreactive score (IRS) as described in previous studies [8, 9]. Based on the IRS score, VEGF staining intensity was divided into four groups as follows: (1) grade 0 (–), IRS 0–3; (2) grade 1 (+), IRS 4–6; (3) grade 2 (++), IRS 7–9; (4) grade 3 (+++), IRS 10–12. For IRS evaluation, ten visual fields from different areas were recorded.

Statistics

All the data in this study were evaluated using SAS software (version 9.1, SAS Institute Inc., Cary, N.C., USA). Differences were considered significant at values of $p < 0.05$. Fisher's exact tests or χ^2 test was used for the analysis of relationships between the expressions of E-cadherin or VEGF, and clinicopathological characters. Cumulative disease-free survival (DFS) was computed using the Kaplan-Meier method and compared between groups by the log-rank test. DFS was measured from the date of liver surgery to the date when recurrent disease was diagnosed or, in the absence of detectable tumor, to the date of death or the last follow-up. To elucidate the relationship between each expression and metastatic recurrence, we also analyzed the hazard ratios (HR) of recurrence within 2 years for each patient group, which were classified according to the intensity of immunohistochemical staining. Using the Cox proportional hazards regression model, HR and 95% CI were calculated and each analysis was performed so as to compare different groups (i.e. metastatic recurrence vs. multicentric recurrence, and multicentric recurrence vs. recurrence-free).

Results

Correlation between E-Cadherin Expression in Noncancerous Liver and Clinical Outcome

E-cadherin staining was specifically observed at the cell boundary. Negative E-cadherin expression was observed more frequently in patients with metastatic recurrence (32.4%; 24/74) than in patients with multicentric recurrence (13.6%; 3/22) or recurrence-free (13.5%; 5/37).

Table 1 compares HR for patients between metastatic recurrence versus multicentric recurrence and recurrence-free and multicentric recurrence versus recurrence-

Table 1. Univariate and multivariate Cox proportional analyses

a Factors associated with metastatic recurrence (metastatic recurrence vs. multicentric carcinoma and recurrence-free)

Variable	Univariate			Multivariate		
	HR	95% CI	p	HR	95% CI	p
Platelet count, $10^3/mm^3$						
$\geq 10 \times 10^4$	1.00		–			
$<10 \times 10^4$	1.30	1.03–1.64	0.029	1.31	1.05–1.68	0.017
E-cadherin expression in noncancerous liver						
Positive	1.00					
Weak positive	1.04	0.79–1.37	0.076			
Negative	1.41	1.06–1.87	0.020	1.43	1.10–1.84	0.009
VEGF expression in noncancerous liver						
Negative	1.00					
Grade 1	1.20	0.82–1.65	0.210			
Grade 2 or Grade 3	1.43	1.02–2.03	0.038			

The patients with grade 3 and grade 2 expression of VEGF in noncancerous tissues are combined for statistical analysis.

b Factors associated with multicentric carcinoma (multicentric carcinoma vs. recurrence-free)

Variable	Univariate			Multivariate		
	HR	95% CI	p	HR	95% CI	p
Hepatitis status			–			
Non-B non-C	1.00					
HCV	1.91	1.16–3.57	0.010	1.83	1.11–3.25	0.017
HBV	0.80	0.18–2.08	0.671			
Clinical stage						
I	1.00		–			
II	1.76	1.10–2.78	0.020			
ALT, IU/l						
≤80	1.00		–			
>80	1.58	1.03–2.45	0.035	1.59	1.03–2.48	0.037

p values were calculated for continuous values by ANOVA and for categorical values for the χ^2 test or Fisher's exact test.

The patients with incomplete data were excluded.

Non-B non-C hepatitis = Negative for hepatitis B surface antigen (HBsAg) and hepatitis C virus antibody (HCVAb) or RNA (–); HCV = positive for HCVAb or HCV-RNA; HBV = positive for HBsAg.

free. These comparisons were made in relation to clinicopathological data from univariate and multivariate analyses, which were performed to evaluate variables that could affect metastatic recurrence or the emergence of multicentric recurrence after curative surgery. According to univariate and multivariate analyses, negative E-cadherin expression in noncancerous liver was associated with increased risk for metastatic recurrence (p = 0.020, HR 1.41, 95% CI 1.06–1.87; p = 0.009, HR 1.43, 95% CI 1.10–1.84 by univariate and multivariate analyses, respectively; table 1). However, no significant relationship existed between multicentric recurrence and expression of E-cadherin by both univariate and multivariate analyses.

Correlation between VEGF Expression in Noncancerous Liver and Clinical Outcome

The proportion of HCC exhibiting grade 2 or 3 expression of VEGF in noncancerous liver was significantly higher in patients with metastatic recurrence (28.4%; 21/74) than those with multicentric recurrence (9.1%; 2/22) or as recurrence-free (10.8%; 4/37, p = 0.038). All cases of grade 3 VEGF expression, even though the number was only 2 patients, experienced metastatic recurrence (100%; 2/2).

For the onset of metastatic recurrence, the degree of VEGF staining in noncancerous liver was significantly correlated with an increased HR for grade 2 or grade 3 expression (p = 0.038, HR 1.43, 95% CI 1.02–2.03) than grade 1 (p = 0.210, HR 1.20, 95% CI 0.82–1.65) by univariate analysis; however, there was no correlation with multivariate analysis (table 1). On the contrary, no significant relationship was observed between VEGF expression and multicentric recurrence.

Clinical Features of the Patients and Outcome

For metastatic recurrence, low platelet count ($<10 \times 10^4$) was revealed to be the significant correlation in both univariate and multivariate analyses (p = 0.029, HR 1.30, 95% CI 1.03–1.64; p = 0.017, HR 1.31, 95% CI 1.05–1.68 by univariate and multivariate analyses, respectively). For multicentric recurrence, the positive for hepatitis C virus antibody (p = 0.010, HR 1.91, 95% CI 1.16–3.57), advanced clinical stage of HCC (p = 0.020, HR 1.76, 95% CI 1.10–2.78) and serum ALT level (>80; p = 0.035, HR 1.58, 95% CI 1.03–2.45) were revealed as significant risk factors in univariate analysis, and the presence of hepatitis C virus and serum ALT level were the independent prognostic factors for emergence of multicentric recurrence by multivariate analysis (p = 0.017, HR = 1.83, 95% CI 1.11–3.25; p = 0.037, HR 1.59, 95% CI 1.03–2.48, respectively; table 1).

DFS of HCC, and Expression of E-Cadherin and VEGF in Noncancerous Liver

The median duration of DFS in patients with multicentric recurrence was significantly longer (87.3 ± 56.7 months) than in patients with metastatic recurrence (22.9 ± 20.5 months; p < 0.001). Negative E-cadherin expres-

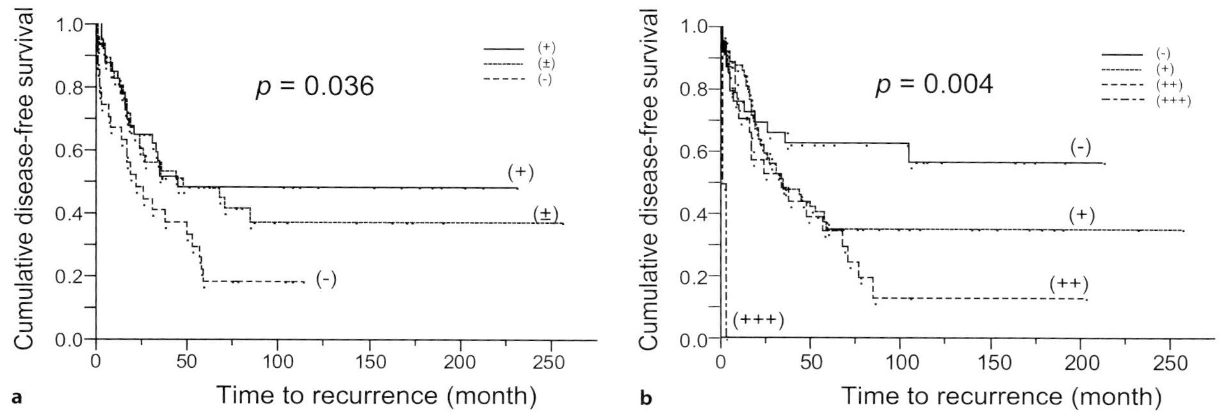

Fig. 1. Comparison of cumulative postoperative DFS curves according to intensity of immunohistochemistry. E-cadherin expression in noncancerous tissue (**a**) and VEGF expression in noncancerous tissue (**b**). Immunostaining intensity was evaluated by the Kaplan-Meier method. The group with negative (–) E-cadherin expression in noncancerous liver tissues exhibited shorter periods of DFS than those with weak positive (±) or positive (+) expression (p = 0.036 by log-rank test). All patients with grade 3 (+++) expression of VEGF in noncancerous tissues exhibited recurrence within 2 years. The group with grade 1 (+), grade 2 (++) or grade 3 (+++) expression of VEGF in noncancerous liver tissues exhibited higher recurrence rates than those with negative (–) expression of VEGF (p = 0.004 by log-rank test).

sion in noncancerous liver correlated with reduced time of DFS, and the recurrence rate correlated negatively with the extent of E-cadherin expression (p = 0.036; fig. 1a). Moreover, HR of recurrence within 2 years for negative E-cadherin expression was higher than the normal expression, although not statistically significant.

All patients with grade 3 for VEGF expression occurred recurrence within 2 years, and HR of recurrence within 2 years was much higher in grade 3 VEGF expression than the other groups (p = 0.004, HR 4.68, 95% CI 1.78–9.70). Furthermore, patients with grade 2 or 3 VEGF expression exhibited higher recurrence rates than those with negative VEGF expression (p = 0.030, HR 2.05, 95% CI 1.04–4.11). The reduced DFS was positively correlated with degree of VEGF expression in noncancerous liver (p = 0.004; fig. 1b).

Discussion

Surgical resection offers good overall survival for patients with HCC [10], although recurrence rates remain high [11]. In the cases of multicentric recurrence, surgical resection of tumor [12], radiofrequency ablation [13] and transplantation [1, 14] should be effective for treatment of recurrent tumor; however, there are few effective treatment options for patients with metastasis. In this study, we found an interesting association between expression of E-cadherin in noncancerous liver and occurrence of metastatic recurrence after curative resection of HCC.

The mechanism of metastasis is, as yet, not fully understood. Increasing evidence suggests that the role of the microenvironment surrounding metastasis appears critical for 'self-seeding' of cancer cells [15, 16], evaluating the 'soil' (premetastatic niche) seems to play an important role for establishment of metastasis. Nonetheless, the relationship between the status of adjacent nontumor liver tissue and metastatic recurrence has not been clarified yet. In this study we focused on the relationship between the supporting noncancerous liver tissue and recurrence signature after curative resection of HCC. It is clear that EMT is involved in metastatic events in cancer [4], besides which, reduced E-cadherin expression is one of the EMT markers [17, 18]. We observed a positive relationship between metastatic recurrence and reduced E-cadherin expression in adjacent noncancerous liver (table 1). For this finding, it is possible to speculate over the two possible roles of E-cadherin expression in the liver. First, reduced E-cadherin in adjacent nontumor liver is associated with presence of microvascular invasion or micrometastasis of primary tumor at the time of surgery. Second, noncancerous liver with reduced E-cadherin expression might be suitable for homing of HCC cells in the circulation, which might lead to loosening of cell-cell contacts of epithelium [19, 20]. In chronic hepatitis and liver cirrhosis, downregulation of E-cadherin by aberrant DNA methylation has been reported [21]. Therefore, epigenetic inactivation of E-cadherin in noncancerous liver might be a risk of metastatic recurrence after curative resection of HCC. Our result also revealed that the only clinical independent factor for predicting emergence of metastatic recurrence was reduced platelet count.

Moreover, we observed that reduced E-cadherin expressions as well as increased VEGF expressions in noncancerous liver were associated with the shorter periods of DFS (fig. 1a, b). It is reported that reduced E-cadherin was associated with increases in HIF-1α and VEGF expression, and elevated microvessel density [22]. Therefore, reduced E-cadherin and increased VEGF expression should be correlated with each other and this association seems to be one of the hallmarks of metastasis in the context of status of background noncancerous liver of HCC. From this standpoint, blocking reductions or improving the expression of E-cadherin might have potential therapeutic implications by suppressing invasiveness and inhibiting the formation of HCC metastases [23].

The IHC expression profiles of E-cadherin in adjacent noncancerous liver tissue revealed high-risk patterns of metastatic recurrence. These results could suggest a promising approach to suppression of metastasis for patients with high risk of postoperative recurrence whose tumors are completely resected.

Disclosure Statement

The authors have no competing interests to declare. This work was supported in part by a grant from the Smoking Research Foundation.

References

1 Poon RT, Fan ST, Lo CM, Liu CL, Wong J: Long-term survival and pattern of recurrence after resection of small hepatocellular carcinoma in patients with preserved liver function: implications for a strategy of salvage transplantation. Ann Surg 2002;235:373–382.
2 Kumada T, Nakano S, Takeda I, Sugiyama K, Osada T, Kiriyama S, Sone Y, Toyoda H, Shimada S, Takahashi M, Sassa T: Patterns of recurrence after initial treatment in patients with small hepatocellular carcinoma. Hepatology 1997;25:87–92.
3 Gupta R: Building patient confidence through effective communication. Br J Hosp Med (Lond) 2006;67:M2–M4.
4 Thiery JP, Acloque H, Huang RY, Nieto MA: Epithelial-mesenchymal transitions in development and disease. Cell 2009;139:871–890.
5 Lyden D, Hattori K, Dias S, Costa C, Blaikie P, Butros L, Chadburn A, Heissig B, Marks W, Witte L, Wu Y, Hicklin D, Zhu Z, Hackett NR, Crystal RG, Moore MA, Hajjar KA, Manova K, Benezra R, Rafii S: Impaired recruitment of bone-marrow-derived endothelial and hematopoietic precursor cells blocks tumor angiogenesis and growth. Nat Med 2001;7:1194–1201.
6 Liver Cancer Study Group of Japan: The general rules for the clinical and pathological study of primary liver cancer. Jpn J Surg 1989;19:98–129.
7 Ikeda K, Arase Y, Kobayashi M, Saitoh S, Someya T, Hosaka T, Suzuki Y, Suzuki F, Tsubota A, Akuta N, Kumada H: Significance of multicentric cancer recurrence after potentially curative ablation of hepatocellular carcinoma: a long-term cohort study of 892 patients with viral cirrhosis. J Gastroenterol 2003;38:865–876.
8 Chui X, Egami H, Yamashita J, Kurizaki T, Ohmachi H, Yamamoto S, Ogawa M: Immunohistochemical expression of the c-kit proto-oncogene product in human malignant and non-malignant breast tissues. Br J Cancer 1996;73:1233–1236.
9 Friedrichs K, Gluba S, Eidtmann H, Jonat W: Overexpression of p53 and prognosis in breast cancer. Cancer 1993;72:3641–3647.
10 Belghiti J, Fuks D: Liver resection and transplantation in hepatocellular carcinoma. Liver Cancer 2012;1:71–82.
11 Lim KC, Chow PK, Allen JC, Siddiqui FJ, Chan ES, Tan SB: Systematic review of outcomes of liver resection for early hepatocellular carcinoma within the Milan criteria. Br J Surg 2012;99:1622–1629.
12 Minagawa M, Makuuchi M, Takayama T, Kokudo N: Selection criteria for repeat hepatectomy in patients with recurrent hepatocellular carcinoma. Ann Surg 2003;238:703–710.
13 Cho YK, Rhim H, Noh S: Radiofrequency ablation versus surgical resection as primary treatment of hepatocellular carcinoma meeting the Milan criteria: a systematic review. J Gastroenterol Hepatol 2011;26:1354–1360.
14 Cheah YL, Chow P: Liver transplantation for heptatocellular carcinoma: an appraisal of the current controversies. Liver Cancer, in press.
15 Erler JT, Bennewith KL, Cox TR, Lang G, Bird D, Koong A, Le QT, Giaccia AJ: Hypoxia-induced lysyl oxidase is a critical mediator of bone marrow cell recruitment to form the premetastatic niche. Cancer Cell 2009;15:35–44.
16 Valastyan S, Weinberg RA: Tumor metastasis: molecular insights and evolving paradigms. Cell 2011;147:275–292.
17 Schmalhofer O, Brabletz S, Brabletz T: E-cadherin, beta-catenin, and ZEB1 in malignant progression of cancer. Cancer Metastasis Rev 2009;28:151–166.
18 Onder TT, Gupta PB, Mani SA, Yang J, Lander ES, Weinberg RA: Loss of E-cadherin promotes metastasis via multiple downstream transcriptional pathways. Cancer Res 2008;68:3645–3654.
19 Paschos KA, Canovas D, Bird NC: The role of cell adhesion molecules in the progression of colorectal cancer and the development of liver metastasis. Cell Signal 2009;21:665–674.
20 Ramis-Conde I, Chaplain MA, Anderson AR, Drasdo D: Multi-scale modelling of cancer cell intravasation: the role of cadherins in metastasis. Phys Biol 2009;6:016008.
21 Kanai Y, Ushijima S, Tsuda H, Sakamoto M, Hirohashi S: Aberrant DNA methylation precedes loss of heterozygosity on chromosome 16 in chronic hepatitis and liver cirrhosis. Cancer Lett 2000;148:73–80.
22 Calvisi DF, Ladu S, Conner EA, Factor VM, Thorgeirsson SS: Disregulation of E-cadherin in transgenic mouse models of liver cancer. Lab Invest 2004;84:1137–1147.
23 Fransvea E, Angelotti U, Antonaci S, Giannelli G: Blocking transforming growth factor-beta up-regulates E-cadherin and reduces migration and invasion of hepatocellular carcinoma cells. Hepatology 2008;47:1557–1566.

Oncology

Oncology 2013;84(suppl 1):93–97
DOI: 10.1159/000345897

Published online: February 20, 2013

Recent Advancements in Comprehensive Genetic Analyses for Human Hepatocellular Carcinoma

Naoshi Nishida   Masatoshi Kudo

Department of Gastroenterology and Hepatology, Kinki University Faculty of Medicine, Osakasayama, Japan

Key Words
Hepatocellular carcinoma · Whole-genome sequencing · Exome analysis · Genome-wide association study

Abstract
Hepatocellular carcinoma (HCC) typically develops in the liver with chronic hepatitis and cirrhosis, and activation of oncogenes and inactivation of tumor suppressor genes occurs during carcinogenesis via genetic and epigenetic mechanisms. Recent advancements in the development of analyses for examining the cancer genome have revealed information regarding genetic alterations in HCC tissues. According to previous studies, the incidence of recurrent genetic alterations in individual genes was thought to be relatively rare and limited to a subset of a few cancer-specific genes such as tumor suppressor *p53*, *RB* genes and oncogenes such as *CTNNB1*. However, recent whole-genome analyses and exome sequencing of tumor DNA have revealed numerous novel alterations of cancer-related genes and pathways critical for HCC development. In addition, various risk factors for HCC, such as the presence or absence of hepatitis B and C virus, may affect the mutation profile of the corresponding cancer genome. On the other hand, genome-wide association studies have also identified important single-nucleotide polymorphisms involved in HCC development, which may allow detection of a group at high risk of HCC emergence. Such analyses will clarify how this malignancy can be treated, diagnosed and prevented more effectively.

Introduction

Hepatocellular carcinoma (HCC) is one of the most common cancers worldwide, and multiple risk factors, such as chronic infection of hepatitis B virus and hepatitis C virus (HCV), alcohol intake and exposure to carcinogens such as aflatoxin B1 are known to be involved in the development of this disease [1]. Thus far, several studies have examined the analytical methods used for determining the molecular characteristics of HCC [2–8]. However, because of the limited number of genes and genomic regions analyzed, genomic alterations and critical pathways involved during hepatocarcinogenesis remains unclear. In contrast, a recent report involving whole-genome and exome analyses of human HCC revealed a novel landscape of genetic alterations, which had not been previously recognized [9, 10]. In this review, we focus on the recent exome analysis and whole-genome DNA sequencing of HCC tissues. We also dis-

KARGER

Fax +41 61 306 12 34
E-Mail karger@karger.com
www.karger.com

0030–2414/13/0847–0093$38.00/0

Accessible online at:
www.karger.com/ocl

Naoshi Nishida, MD
Department of Gastroenterology and Hepatology
Kinki University Faculty of Medicine
377-2 Ohno-higashi, Osakasayama, Osaka 589-8511 (Japan)
E-Mail naoshi@med.kindai.ac.jp

cuss a genome-wide association study (GWAS) involving the somatic cells of HCC patients, which revealed critical single-nucleotide polymorphisms (SNPs) important for identifying patients at high risk of HCC emergence [11].

Base Substitution and Etiology of HCC

A profile of base substitutions resulting in mutations in HCC has been reported on the basis of mutation analyses of the tumor suppressor *TP53* gene, in which G>T/C>A transversions were predominant [2, 12]. Most base substitutions were detected on the nontranscribed strand, which may be attributed to preferential repair of the transcribed strand [2]. Further, aflatoxin B1 is known to induce G>T/C>A transversions at codon 249, and many HCCs in China and South Africa reportedly carry this mutation [12, 13]. Recently, Guichard et al. [14] performed whole-exome sequencing and reported that G>T/C>A transversions were significantly more frequent in tumors that developed on noncirrhotic liver. This suggests that specific genotoxic agents, such as aflatoxin B1, may contribute in part to HCC emergence without the background condition of liver cirrhosis. Most HCC cases in this cohort were in patients from France and not likely associated with aflatoxin B1; therefore, another genotoxin may be involved in HCC carcinogenesis [14]. Substitutions of G>T/C>A and T>A>A>T transversions were also frequently detected in HBV-related HCCs with portal vein thrombosis (PVTT) [15].

In contrast, Totoki et al. [16] performed a massive parallel sequencing of HCV-positive HCC and found a predominance of T>C/A>G substitutions at the ApT site in the genomes of HCV-related HCCs compared to smoking- and ultraviolet-related cancers. A study by Fujimoto et al. [17] showed that the C>T/G>A at the CpG site was also important. However, because this type of transition was also predominant in other cancers, they concluded that T>C/A>G and C>A/G>T substitutions may be characteristic of HCCs in Japan, where most HCCs were HCV-related [17]. They also reported that habitual alcohol consumption and occurrence of synchronous or metachronous multiple liver nodules were significantly associated with components of the somatic substitution profile of HCC [17]. Therefore, variations in somatic substitution patterns in HCCs may reflect a difference in status of hepatitis virus and exposure to various carcinogens.

Mutational Profile of Cancer-Related Genes and Etiology of HCC

By analyzing HCV-related HCCs, several somatic mutations have been reported, including the *TP53*, *AXIN1*, *ADAM22*, *JAK2*, *KHDRBS2*, *NEK8* and *TRRAP* genes, as well as a large number of somatic mutations in genes encoding phosphoproteins and those with bipartite nuclear signals [16]. Through high-resolution characterization, they also identified intratumor heterogeneity of the mutations, including inactivation of the *TSC* complex in a subpopulation of the tumors [16]. Li et al. [18] also reported differences in mutated genes among HCCs with several etiologies, focusing on 5 genes: *ARID2*, *CTNNB1*, *TP53*, *DMXL1* and *NLRP1*. Mutations in the *ARID2* gene, which encodes a subunit of the chromatin remodeling complex, were more frequently detected in HCV-related HCC compared with HBV-related HCC [18]. In addition, mutations in the *ARID2* gene were correlated with *CTNNB1* mutations and were mutually exclusive with *TP53* mutations [18]. *CTNNB1* mutations were also more frequently observed in HCV-related HCCs than in HBV-related tumors. In contrast, the prevalence of *TP53* mutations was significantly higher in patients from China [18], where HBV infection is the leading cause of hepatocarcinogenesis.

Huang et al. [19] performed RNA sequence analysis of HBV-related HCC and identified a novel, highly unregulated exon-exon junction in the *ATAD2* gene. According to high-resolution copy number analysis and whole genome sequencing, novel recurrent alterations in the *ARID1A*, *RPS6KA3*, *NFE2L2* and *IRF2* genes were detected [14]. Interestingly, inactivation of the *IRF2* gene was exclusively observed in HBV-related HCC, which led to disruption of *TP53* function [14]. However, mutations in chromatin remodelers were observed in association with alcohol-related HCC [14]. They also reported an association between highly rearranged copy number profile and HCC progression, such as high serum tumor markers, larger size and tumor dedifferentiation [14], which was suggested previously [20, 21]. Further, a high degree of copy number alterations was more frequently observed in HBV-related tumor, tumors developed in noncirrhotic liver and tumors with the *TP53* mutation [14, 22]. They described the 5 major pathways commonly altered by somatic mutations and homozygous deletions, including the Wnt/beta-catenin, p53/cell cycle control, chromatin remodeling, PI3K/Ras signaling and oxidative and endoplasmic reticulum stress pathways. Among these, the Wnt/beta-catenin pathway was the most frequently altered pathway according to whole-genome sequencing [14]. This study also revealed that most *CTNNB1* mutations were present in tumors without HBV infection and were mutually exclusive to the*TP53* mutation [14], which is consistent with the results of Li et al. [18]. In contrast, mutations in the *AXIN1* and *APC* genes were detected in tumors with various etiologies and showed no relationship with*TP53* mutations. Alterations in *IRF2*, which is involved in the p53 pathway, are associated with HBV infection and high chromosomal instability [14]. Mutations of the chromatin remodeling-related genes *ARID1A* were significantly more frequent in alcohol-related HCC and showed an association with the *CTNNB1* mutation [14]. Overall, >24% of HCCs possessed mutations in at least one of the genes involved in the chromatin remodeling pathway. Mutations of the *RPS6KA3* gene, which encodes a component involved in PI3K/Ras signaling, were detected predominantly in HCC without cirrhosis and associated with *AXIN1* mutations [14]. Mutations in the *NFE2L2* gene, which encodes a component of the oxidative and endoplasmic reticulum stress pathways, showed an association with alterations in the Wnt/beta-catenin pathway [14].

Fujimoto et al. [17] also analyzed HCC with various etiologies and showed that 52% of HCCs carried mutations in at least one of the genes associated with chromatin regulation, including *ARID1A*, *ARID1B*, *ARID2*, *MLL*, *MLL3*, *BAZ2B*, *BRD8*, *BPTF*, *BRE* and *HIST1H4B*. These mutations were marginally associated with the stage of liver fibrosis and hepatic invasion. Huang et al. [15] also analyzed HBV-related HCC with PVTT and intrahepatic metastasis by using exome sequencing. The gene that encodes the component of the chromatin remodeling complex, *ARID1A*, was mutated in 13% of subjects in the HBV-related HCC cohort [15]. However, mutations in this gene were also observed in HCV-related and non-virus-infected HCCs. They also described that mutations in *VCAM1* and *TMEM35* genes may be potential driver mutations for hepatocarcinogenesis [15].

Integration of HBV Genome into Host DNA

For HCC cases with HBV infection, HBV integration was reportedly observed within or upstream of the *TERT* gene in tumor tissues [17]. Recurrent integration of HBV was also detected in the *FAR2*, *ITPR1*, *IRAK2*, *MAPK1*, *MLL* and *MLL4* genes [23–26]. In addition to integration of HBV into the *TERT* gene, Sung et al. [27] reported integration events at the *MLL4* and *CCNE1*, and *SENP5* and *ROCK1* genes. They found that most HBV breakpoints in HCC were close to active coding genes, potentially allowing HBV to integrate into the open chromatin region more effectively [27]. Breakpoints in HBV were over-represented in exon and promoter in HCC issues, but these were primarily detected in introns in noncancerous liver tissues, which may be attributed to positive selective pressure induced by integration of HBV into exons and promoters of active genes [27].

Jiang et al. [28] also performed comprehensive analyses of HBV-related HCC and their corresponding normal tissues using Alu-PCR, ligation-mediated PCR and an array-based comparative genomic hybridization assay. Nontumor liver tissues carried many viral integration sites randomly scattered throughout the genome. However, clonal and high-abundance viral integrations were detected in tumor tissue [27, 28]. Integration events may lead to abnormal expression of genes close to the integration sites, emergence of fusion genes and alterations of DNA copy number [28], which has also been suggested in another study [27].

A larger number of HBV integration events is reportedly associated with a high serum level of hepatitis surface antigen, α-fetoprotein, younger age of HCC emergence and chromosome copy number [14, 27]. Interestingly, it is also associated with patient survival and tumor aggressiveness [27].

Evolution of Genetic Alteration during Tumor Progression

Whole-genome sequencing is a powerful tool that can be used to identify candidate driver mutations of carcinogenesis using human tissue samples. Tao et al. [29] analyzed the evolution of HCC using 9 different sections of 3 tumors, including original and metastatic lesions and 7 sections of adjacent nontumor tissues by using whole-genome sequencing. In these analyses, somatic mutations were used to define 4 evolutionary linkages among tumor cells and candidate diver mutations of tumor progression of these HCC cases were speculated. Huang et al. [15] compared primary tumors and their PVTT lesions and reported that 94.2% of mutations were identical among primary tumors and PVTT. However, PVTT cases are thought to be derived from primary tumors, and mutations in the *KDM6A* and *CUL9* genes were exclusively detected in PVTT, suggesting that these mutations play a role in tumor progression [15].

Genetic Risk of HCC

Although hepatitis virus infection, alcohol consumption, obesity, diabetes mellitus and intake of genotoxic agents such as aflatoxin B1 are known critical risk factors for developing HCC, genetic factors determined on the basis of the nucleotide sequence of the host genome may also play a role in malignancy [11]. Several reports have suggested the association between polymorphisms in individual genes and the risk of HCC. For example, SNPs of the *SCBY14*, *CRHR2*, *GFRA1*, *CCND2*, *RAD23B*, *GRP78*, *CEP164*, *MDM2* and *ALDH2* genes were reportedly associated with an increased risk of HCC in Japanese patients with HCV infection [30, 31].

Recently, a GWAS revealed that intronic SNPs in the *DEPDC5* locus on chromosome 22 are associated with HCC risk in Japanese patients with chronic hepatitis C [32]. The *DEPDC5* gene is known to be involved in bladder carcinogenesis, but the function of this gene remains debatable [33]. Kumar et al. [34] also performed a GWAS on HCV-related HCCs and found a novel SNP of rs2596542 located in the 5′-region of the *MICA* gene on chromosome 6p. According to the GWAS conducted to identify risk of HBV-related hepatocarcinogenesis, an intronic SNP of the *KIF1B* gene on chromosome 1p was reported, and SNPs in the *UBE4B* and *PGD* genes were also shown to be significant for HCC emergence among HBV-positive patients [35].

Conclusion

Through comprehensive and precise analyses of cancer genomes, novel mutations and alterations in individual pathways involved in HCC development have been clarified. This information may be critical for establishing novel biomarkers for cancer therapy. Furthermore, these analyses will provide useful information for developing novel molecular-targeted therapy of this refractory cancer. Also, GWAS using DNA of somatic cells will be important for specifically identifying those at high risk of developing HCC. Accumulation of genetic information regarding cancer and somatic cells may help clarify how HCC should be managed to prevent HCC more effectively in the future.

Disclosure Statement

The authors have no competing interests to declare. This work was supported in part by a grant from the Smoking Research Foundation.

References

1 Kim DY, Han K: Epidemiology and surveilance of hepatocellular carcinoma. Liver Cancer 2012;1:2–14.
2 Nishida N, Fukuda Y, Kokuryu H, Toguchida J, Yandell DW, Ikenega M, Imura H, Ishizaki K: Role and mutational heterogeneity of the p53 gene in hepatocellular carcinoma. Cancer Res 1993;53:368–372.
3 Nishida N, Fukuda Y, Komeda T, Kita R, Sando T, Furukawa M, Amenomori M, Shibagaki I, Nakao K, Ikenaga M, et al: Amplification and overexpression of the cyclin D1 gene in aggressive human hepatocellular carcinoma. Cancer Res 1994;54:3107–3110.
4 Nishida N, Fukuda Y, Ishizaki K, Nakao K: Alteration of cell cycle-related genes in hepatocarcinogenesis. Histol Histopathol 1997; 12:1019–1025.
5 Nishida N, Nishimura T, Ito T, Komeda T, Fukuda Y, Nakao K: Chromosomal instability and human hepatocarcinogenesis. Histol Histopathol 2003;18:897–909.
6 Nishida N, Nagasaka T, Nishimura T, Ikai I, Boland CR, Goel A: Aberrant methylation of multiple tumor suppressor genes in aging liver, chronic hepatitis, and hepatocellular carcinoma. Hepatology 2008;47:908–918.
7 Nishida N: Impact of hepatitis virus and aging on DNA methylation in human hepatocarcinogenesis. Histol Histopathol 2010;25: 647–654.
8 Nishida N, Goel A: Genetic and epigenetic signatures in human hepatocellular carcinoma: a systematic review. Curr Genomics 2011;12:130–137.
9 Toffanin S, Cornella H, Harrington A, Llovet JM: Next-generation sequencing: path for driver discovery in hepatocellular carcinoma. Gastroenterology 2012;143:1391–1393.
10 Zhang Z: Genomic landscape of liver cancer. Nat Genet 2012;44:1075–1077.
11 Hoshida Y, Fuchs BC, Tanabe KK: Genomic risk of hepatitis C-related hepatocellular carcinoma. J Hepatol 2012;56:729–730.
12 Hsu IC, Metcalf RA, Sun T, Welsh JA, Wang NJ, Harris CC: Mutational hotspot in the p53 gene in human hepatocellular carcinomas. Nature 1991;350:427–428.
13 Bressac B, Kew M, Wands J, Ozturk M: Selective G to T mutations of p53 gene in hepatocellular carcinoma from southern Africa. Nature 1991;350:429–431.
14 Guichard C, Amaddeo G, Imbeaud S, Ladeiro Y, Pelletier L, Maad IB, Calderaro J, Bioulac-Sage P, Letexier M, Degos F, Clement B, Balabaud C, Chevet E, Laurent A, Couchy G, Letouze E, Calvo F, Zucman-Rossi J: Integrated analysis of somatic mutations and focal copy-number changes identifies key genes and pathways in hepatocellular carcinoma. Nat Genet 2012;44:694–698.
15 Huang J, Deng Q, Wang Q, Li KY, Dai JH, Li N, Zhu ZD, Zhou B, Liu XY, Liu RF, Fei QL, Chen H, Cai B, Xiao HS, Qin LX, Han ZG: Exome sequencing of hepatitis B virus-associated hepatocellular carcinoma. Nat Genet 2012;44:1117–1121.

16 Totoki Y, Tatsuno K, Yamamoto S, Arai Y, Hosoda F, Ishikawa S, Tsutsumi S, Sonoda K, Totsuka H, Shirakihara T, Sakamoto H, Wang L, Ojima H, Shimada K, Kosuge T, Okusaka T, Kato K, Kusuda J, Yoshida T, Aburatani H, Shibata T: High-resolution characterization of a hepatocellular carcinoma genome. Nat Genet 2011;43:464–469.
17 Fujimoto A, Totoki Y, Abe T, Boroevich KA, Hosoda F, Nguyen HH, Aoki M, Hosono N, Kubo M, Miya F, Arai Y, Takahashi H, Shirakihara T, Nagasaki M, Shibuya T, Nakano K, Watanabe-Makino K, Tanaka H, Nakamura H, Kusuda J, Ojima H, Shimada K, Okusaka T, Ueno M, Shigekawa Y, Kawakami Y, Arihiro K, Ohdan H, Gotoh K, Ishikawa O, Ariizumi S, Yamamoto M, Yamada T, Chayama K, Kosuge T, Yamaue H, Kamatani N, Miyano S, Nakagama H, Nakamura Y, Tsunoda T, Shibata T, Nakagawa H: Whole-genome sequencing of liver cancers identifies etiological influences on mutation patterns and recurrent mutations in chromatin regulators. Nat Genet 2012;44:760–764.
18 Li M, Zhao H, Zhang X, Wood LD, Anders RA, Choti MA, Pawlik TM, Daniel HD, Kannangai R, Offerhaus GJ, Velculescu VE, Wang L, Zhou S, Vogelstein B, Hruban RH, Papadopoulos N, Cai J, Torbenson MS, Kinzler KW: Inactivating mutations of the chromatin remodeling gene ARID2 in hepatocellular carcinoma. Nat Genet 2011;43: 828–829.
19 Huang Q, Lin B, Liu H, Ma X, Mo F, Yu W, Li L, Li H, Tian T, Wu D, Shen F, Xing J, Chen ZN: RNA-Seq analyses generate comprehensive transcriptomic landscape and reveal complex transcript patterns in hepatocellular carcinoma. PLoS One 2011;6:e26168.
20 Nishida N, Fukuda Y, Kokuryu H, Sadamoto T, Isowa G, Honda K, Yamaoka Y, Ikenaga M, Imura H, Ishizaki K: Accumulation of allelic loss on arms of chromosomes 13q, 16q and 17p in the advanced stages of human hepatocellular carcinoma. Int J Cancer 1992;51: 862–868.
21 Nishida N, Fukuda Y, Komeda T, Ito T, Nishimura T, Minata M, Kuno M, Katsuma H, Ikai I, Yamaoka Y, Nakao K: Prognostic impact of multiple allelic losses on metastatic recurrence in hepatocellular carcinoma after curative resection. Oncology 2002;62: 141–148.
22 Nishida N, Nishimura T, Nagasaka T, Ikai I, Goel A, Boland CR: Extensive methylation is associated with beta-catenin mutations in hepatocellular carcinoma: evidence for two distinct pathways of human hepatocarcinogenesis. Cancer Res 2007;67:4586–4594.
23 Gozuacik D, Murakami Y, Saigo K, Chami M, Mugnier C, Lagorce D, Okanoue T, Urashima T, Brechot C, Paterlini-Brechot P: Identification of human cancer-related genes by naturally occurring hepatitis B virus DNA tagging. Oncogene 2001;20:6233–6240.
24 Paterlini-Brechot P, Saigo K, Murakami Y, Chami M, Gozuacik D, Mugnier C, Lagorce D, Brechot C: Hepatitis B virus-related insertional mutagenesis occurs frequently in human liver cancers and recurrently targets human telomerase gene. Oncogene 2003;22: 3911–3916.
25 Murakami Y, Saigo K, Takashima H, Minami M, Okanoue T, Brechot C, Paterlini-Brechot P: Large scaled analysis of hepatitis B virus (HBV) DNA integration in HBV related hepatocellular carcinomas. Gut 2005;54: 1162–1168.
26 Saigo K, Yoshida K, Ikeda R, Sakamoto Y, Murakami Y, Urashima T, Asano T, Kenmochi T, Inoue I: Integration of hepatitis B virus DNA into the myeloid/lymphoid or mixed-lineage leukemia (MLL4) gene and rearrangements of MLL4 in human hepatocellular carcinoma. Hum Mutat 2008;29:703–708.
27 Sung WK, Zheng H, Li S, Chen R, Liu X, Li Y, Lee NP, Lee WH, Ariyaratne PN, Tennakoon C, Mulawadi FH, Wong KF, Liu AM, Poon RT, Fan ST, Chan KL, Gong Z, Hu Y, Lin Z, Wang G, Zhang Q, Barber TD, Chou WC, Aggarwal A, Hao K, Zhou W, Zhang C, Hardwick J, Buser C, Xu J, Kan Z, Dai H, Mao M, Reinhard C, Wang J, Luk JM: Genome-wide survey of recurrent HBV integration in hepatocellular carcinoma. Nat Genet 2012; 44:765–769.
28 Jiang S, Yang Z, Li W, Li X, Wang Y, Zhang J, Xu C, Chen PJ, Hou J, McCrae MA, Chen X, Zhuang H, Lu F: Re-evaluation of the carcinogenic significance of hepatitis B virus integration in hepatocarcinogenesis. PLoS One 2012;7:e40363.
29 Tao Y, Ruan J, Yeh SH, Lu X, Wang Y, Zhai W, Cai J, Ling S, Gong Q, Chong Z, Qu Z, Li Q, Liu J, Yang J, Zheng C, Zeng C, Wang HY, Zhang J, Wang SH, Hao L, Dong L, Li W, Sun M, Zou W, Yu C, Li C, Liu G, Jiang L, Xu J, Huang H, Mi S, Zhang B, Chen B, Zhao W, Hu S, Zhuang SM, Shen Y, Shi S, Brown C, White KP, Chen DS, Chen PJ, Wu CI: Rapid growth of a hepatocellular carcinoma and the driving mutations revealed by cell-population genetic analysis of whole-genome data. Proc Natl Acad Sci USA 2011;108:12042–12047.
30 Kato N, Ji G, Wang Y, Baba M, Hoshida Y, Otsuka M, Taniguchi H, Moriyama M, Dharel N, Goto T, Shao RX, Matsuura T, Ishii K, Shiina S, Kawabe T, Muramatsu M, Omata M: Large-scale search of single nucleotide polymorphisms for hepatocellular carcinoma susceptibility genes in patients with hepatitis C. Hepatology 2005;42:846–853.
31 Tomoda T, Nouso K, Sakai A, Ouchida M, Kobayashi S, Miyahara K, Onishi H, Nakamura S, Yamamoto K, Shimizu K: Genetic risk of hepatocellular carcinoma in patients with hepatitis C virus: a case control study. J Gastroenterol Hepatol 2012;27:797–804.
32 Miki D, Ochi H, Hayes CN, Abe H, Yoshima T, Aikata H, Ikeda K, Kumada H, Toyota J, Morizono T, Tsunoda T, Kubo M, Nakamura Y, Kamatani N, Chayama K: Variation in the DEPDC5 locus is associated with progression to hepatocellular carcinoma in chronic hepatitis C virus carriers. Nat Genet 2011;43: 797–800.
33 Kanehira M, Harada Y, Takata R, Shuin T, Miki T, Fujioka T, Nakamura Y, Katagiri T: Involvement of upregulation of DEPDC1 (dep domain containing 1) in bladder carcinogenesis. Oncogene 2007;26:6448–6455.
34 Kumar V, Kato N, Urabe Y, Takahashi A, Muroyama R, Hosono N, Otsuka M, Tateishi R, Omata M, Nakagawa H, Koike K, Kamatani N, Kubo M, Nakamura Y, Matsuda K: Genome-wide association study identifies a susceptibility locus for HCV-induced hepatocellular carcinoma. Nat Genet 2011;43: 455–458.
35 Zhang H, Zhai Y, Hu Z, Wu C, Qian J, Jia W, Ma F, Huang W, Yu L, Yue W, Wang Z, Li P, Zhang Y, Liang R, Wei Z, Cui Y, Xie W, Cai M, Yu X, Yuan Y, Xia X, Zhang X, Yang H, Qiu W, Yang J, Gong F, Chen M, Shen H, Lin D, Zeng YX, He F, Zhou G: Genome-wide association study identifies 1p36.22 as a new susceptibility locus for hepatocellular carcinoma in chronic hepatitis B virus carriers. Nat Genet 2010;42:755–758.

Oncology

Author Index Vol. 84, Suppl. 1, 2013

Subject Index Vol. 84, Suppl. 1, 2013

KARGER
E-Mail karger@karger.com

Accessible online at:
www.karger.com/ocl